MY JOURNEY BACK TO HEALTH

HEALING CANCER WITHOUT CHEMOTHERAPY
OR RADIATION

LESLIE GRAY ROBBINS

DEDICATION

I am so grateful for my husband, West, my daughter, Addison, and my son, Langdon, who have tirelessly supported me through the whole crazy journey, making me laugh and cry, giving me lots of cuddles, and most of all, giving me the strongest reason to meet this challenge head-on and learn how to THRIVE.

I have been blessed with some of the most amazing friends who have stepped up when I so desperately needed them, helping to entertain the kids, keeping my spirits up, and reminding me that I am loved.

My path wasn't typical, but I stayed true to myself. My story is dedicated to all of the amazing people who stood by me, and my individual decisions, every step of the way.

ACKNOWLEDGMENTS

Thank you to Christine Gray for encouraging me to put my story down on paper and seek a publisher. She, and so many others, gave me the courage to put my experiences out there for all to see, in hopes of inspiring patients to put themselves at the forefront of their care.

We all get to make choices every day – choices that either support our health, or create disease.

CHOOSE HEALTH

FOREWORD

Thank you for reading the details of my healing journey, and thank you to those who have reached out to let me know that you've found inspiration in my words. I'm so grateful to be reaching people and hopefully motivating them to make small changes in their own lives, and to consider another perspective of health.

It can be difficult to share such an intimate story, and to relive the ups and downs is both emotional and cathartic. Thank you for letting me share my story with you.

I am especially moved to hear from other Cancer Thrivers and those with loved ones currently on a healing journey. That is my ultimate goal - to connect to others touched by cancer and spread the word that there are other options available. You are not alone.

It was so difficult for us to find a place like Marinus, and it is a shame that it has to be such an uphill challenge to learn about alternatives. We should be presented with all of the possible options so we can each decide for ourselves what is best for us.

Even if you decide the conventional path is right for you, these holistic approaches can help you heal faster, and make some of the dreadful side effects more bearable.

In the end, nobody truly knows what will work and what won't, not even the experts. I've lost so many friends since my journey began - some did conventional treatments, and some did holistic. Cancer is a wicked beast, and there are no guarantees no matter what path we take.

I am a huge believer that the patient, no matter the disease, MUST be an advocate for himself or herself. You must be the captain of your own ship and not give your power to any doctor or well-meaning family member or friend. Only YOU know what feels right for you, and you must take responsibility for your choices.

Take time to get quiet and listen to what your body truly needs. Put together a team of wise people (doctors, healers, friends, etc.) who will support your wishes and respect your boundaries, whatever they may be.

I'm just a typical human being – not particularly bold or strong. I don't want anyone to think that I'm special, or that they'd have to have some amazing strength in order to heal themselves. They simply need to find the courage to listen to their instincts and do what is truly right for them. SO many cancer patients have told me that they're afraid to go against what the doctors say. But we only have one life and we alone get to decide how we live it.

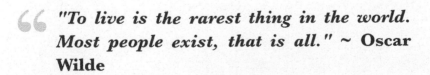 *"To live is the rarest thing in the world. Most people exist, that is all." ~ Oscar Wilde*

THE JOURNEY BEGINS

"We don't know how strong we are until being STRONG is the only choice we have."
~ Author Unknown

Some of you know my story, but many of you don't. It is such a personal thing, but I am neither ashamed of my story nor shy about sharing my health challenges. Saying the word takes the power away from it...

CANCER.

It's a scary word that comes with incredibly scary feelings. But I've found that when you face your fears head on, instead of shying away from the fears, it empowers you.

I recently sent a t-shirt to an old friend of mine who is also dealing with a recent cancer diagnosis, and the words spoke to me: "We don't know how strong we are until being STRONG is the only choice we have" - Truth.

With one phone call, your entire life can change direction. Suddenly, what seemed so important, well, doesn't seem so important after all. Those special moments with your family, those moments by yourself doing something that brings you joy, moments of doing absolutely nothing, or moments of healing – those become the important things that carry such meaning.

All the things that keep us busy every day, things that fill our schedules, and make us feel useful, but don't truly make us happy... they seem almost ridiculous now when facing your own mortality.

I got the call around 4 pm on June 21, 2018.

On the other end of the line was the head of the breast center, and she was certainly lacking in compassion. In a very business-like tone, she said, "So we got your biopsy results, and you have breast cancer. I'll need you to come in next week."

Well, gosh... that's pretty big news to drop on someone, and then expect them to wait almost a week until you give them any details at all. I said, "wait... what does that mean?" I mean, come on – I've never been told I have cancer before, so this was new to me. And as far as I could see, it was a pretty big deal. I could have done with a little kindness - perhaps, "Are you sitting down?" or "Do you have someone with you?"

Nope, it was tossed out there like it was nothing more than, "your tire is low. You'll want to get that fixed soon."

I hung up, feeling completely numb. I was quite sure I didn't want to go see this particular doctor the following week, and most likely never. I have always been the kind of person who needs to connect to my doc – I need to feel cared for. Bedside manner goes a long way in my book, and this lady didn't have it.

So I called my gynecologist, whom I trusted very much. He said it was the 2nd call he'd gotten that day complaining about this particular breast center. Well, at least it wasn't personal.

Within 20 minutes, he had spoken to pathology at the

hospital and gotten all available information on my biopsy results. Thank heavens for Dr. Rock! Truly, I can't say enough wonderful things about him.

Anyway, he told me that I had Invasive Ductal Carcinoma, and it was aggressive – 70+% proliferation rate, which means the cells were dividing and multiplying rapidly.

I could hear the urgency in his voice. He said, "I want you to meet with a breast surgeon whom I trust – I would send my wife to him if she had this diagnosis. And I want you to see him tomorrow, if possible."

He made the call to the surgeon, who was in surgery on Fridays, but was able to get me in on Monday (3 days before I would even be getting my detailed results from the hospital that did the biopsy).

THE FIRST DAYS

"The body can heal itself. Spontaneous healing is not a miracle but a fact of biology – the result of the natural healing system that each one of us is born with." ~ **Dr. Andrew Weil**

The days following the news were a whirl of mixed emotions and confusion. I knew that I wanted to get several opinions on treatments before making the decision that was best for me. I was fortunate to have people in my circle who have been down this road and stepped up to guide me in the most amazing ways.

West and I spent all day Friday, the day after the life-altering call, driving around the suburbs gathering all of my records and images, so we'd have them for the upcoming consults.

One of my dear friends, Caryn, arranged for a 3-way call with her friend from college who had a similar experience 5 years prior. This friend is a wise woman who clearly did her research (in fact, research is her job, so I knew she was thorough), though she was quick to admit that she's learned a lot in the years since her journey, and if she knew then what she knew now, she would have made some different choices.

We had a long conversation over speaker phone while my husband drove down 294, stopping at pathology labs and doctors' offices to gathering various paperwork, images and slides. I never realized how important it was to keep reports from every doctor appointment.

Note: request your paperwork immediately after every appointment and keep all of it in a file, so you have it when needed – even if you don't think you'll need it. I had to jump through hoops to get all of my *own* information from the past 2 decades. It is our right to make those requests – this is YOUR life, and you are entitled to all information about your care. Believe me, it's easier to do it right away than to have to deal with it during a health crisis.

It was fascinating to review all of my mammography results from years past. I learned some things... but more on that later.

I can't remember much of what she said during that conversation, but thankfully my amazing friend was at the ready, taking copious notes as she spoke. She typed them up and emailed them to me later that day. Thank GOD for friends! (You'll hear me say this a lot...)

One of the many important things my fellow Cancer Thriver shared was the name of her surgeon (selected after several consults and much research). I made a note of his name and knew that I'd be requesting a consult with him as well.

She also told us about a documentary called *Cancer Can Be Killed* by Jeff Witzeman that she wished she had seen before having a radical double mastectomy 5 years prior. You can find the documentary here:

www.vimeo.com/ondemand/cancercanbekilled

If she had been aware of the holistic cancer treatments available in countries like Germany at the time of her own diagnosis, she said she would have tried that path first before taking the Western Medicine path. Those were powerful words from a fellow patient who was technically cancer-free 5 years later, but the truth was that it came at a price, and she wasn't shy about sharing the details. I so appreciated her candor.

My head was still spinning, but West was more clear-headed and watched the entire documentary. My very rational husband likes facts and figures and doesn't often let emotion cloud his judgment, so I was surprised when he came to me and said, "This actually makes a lot of sense. I think we should try this path." I knew that I needed to sit down and watch it.

So over the very long weekend filled with work events and family obligations, between the diagnosis and the first consult, I carved out time to sit alone and take it all in.

And then I did my research.

West and I were incredibly intrigued by the idea of holistic cancer treatments. Was it possible to treat the WHOLE patient and not just focus on the tumor or the disease? Could I possibly refuse the 'standard of care' in the U.S., and go against the recommendations of the Western Medicine doctors? The big question was: does it make sense to me - not anyone else, but to ME - to allow my body to be poisoned and burned in order to heal it?

SECOND OPINIONS & THEN SOME

"Perspective may help you see that your chaos is actually just a GIGANTIC blessing."
~ Rachel Hollis

I was busy scheduling several consults with surgeons for the coming week to discuss my case and possible treatment options. If you know me at all, you know I'm not one to sit around and 'wait' for things to happen, and I certainly wasn't going to waste any time when my life literally depended on it.

Now how do you go about finding a cancer specialist you can trust, especially when you're new to this whole 'cancer thing'? You start talking to others and sharing your story.

The initial instinct to keep your diagnosis to yourself is strong, perhaps out of fear of what others might say, or because it's easier to live a 'normal life' if people don't know what you're going through. You have to do what is right and true for you, and only you. However, I will say that in hindsight, I'm very glad I shared my story.

Not long after my diagnosis, I had a miraculous team of over 100 people that buoyed my spirits and resolve by sending me healing vibes and prayers regularly. I don't know where I'd be today without them. I also discovered that the more I shared my journey with others, the more stories came to light, and I realized I wasn't alone. SUPPORT is everything on this journey.

I was a lucky lady indeed.

It might sound weird to say I'm lucky with all that I've been facing, but the truth is that a life-threatening disease quickly puts things into perspective. People and experiences are the things that matter. I was finding reasons to be grateful on a daily basis, and that is a gift. In all honesty, this experience strengthened many of my important relationships. Family and friends stepped up, even when I didn't ask – especially when I didn't ask! It was incredibly humbling...

It's clear that cancer is becoming more prevalent in our world. It is taking hold in people who are far from elderly, myself included. It is not uncommon to see many patients in their 50's, 40's or even 30's at the cancer clinics dealing with their own mortality. Something is wrong with this picture...

It's truly mind-boggling to discover the crazy numbers of people who are on the cancer journey (this journey never truly ends), but the silver lining is that we have each other to lean on. I had a lot of people offering guidance who had been on the cancer journey before me, and I am so grateful for all of them.

A friend and fellow mom currently dealing with a breast cancer diagnosis shared the number of a surgeon nearby with whom she had consulted, so I made an appointment to see that surgeon on Monday afternoon. My cousin had breast cancer many years ago and highly recommended her surgeon in Winfield, so I made an appointment for a consult on the following Wednesday. There was also the surgeon in Glenview who had performed the double mastectomy for my Cancer Thriver friend – I needed to get in there, too.

Monday finally came after a sleepless weekend, and the week of consults and gathering of information and opinions began.

This fellow Cancer Thriver had shared a meticulous document containing a wide range of questions that I should ask any potential surgeon. *Are they familiar with mapping? *Do they believe in nipple sparing? *Would they be sampling nodes? The list of questions went on for 2 pages. These things were all so foreign to me... and it was scary and overwhelming.

And much to my amazement, this incredible person, who really didn't know me very well, offered to meet me at the surgeon's office for my first consult and sit by my side in support. And that's exactly what she did.

She met us at the Lake Forest office of the first surgeon whom we consulted on Monday (Dr. G.), and I can't tell you how helpful it was to have her there, and how incredibly touched I was that she would do this. That she would take time out of her busy day (she is also a working mother and has a lot to juggle) to sit with someone going through a tough time, well, it was very telling of her character and her heart.

DIZZYING CONVERSATIONS

"Everything we hear is an opinion, not a fact.
Everything we see is perspective, not the truth."
~ Marcus Aurelius

So there I sat across from Dr. G., with my husband and my friend by my side, waiting to hear his thoughts on my case. My head was still spinning a bit, and I was incredibly nervous to be in this position, but I couldn't bury my head and pretend it wasn't happening. I needed to do *something,* and quickly. In order to know what the best 'something' for me would be, I needed to gather lots of information.

We would quickly learn that triple negative breast cancer is tricky. All of the surgeons would give me the 'sympathetic head tilt' when they heard that this was the pathology of my particular cancer. You see, triple negative means that this cancer doesn't have any hormone receptors, so there are very limited options for treatment. You can't use the typical hormone therapies that are so often given for breast cancer.

Dr. G. was a kind man who never made us feel rushed. After reviewing my pathology report, he recommended that I have a lumpectomy to remove the tumor as soon as possible, followed by radiation, and then begin a powerful cocktail of 3 different chemotherapy drugs.

I told him that we were considering going to Germany for alternative treatments as we'd heard some amazing stories of healing, and we wanted to get his thoughts. He was skeptical, stating that it's all anecdotal evidence (there are limited studies on natural treatments - truth be told, clinical trials are incredibly expensive, and nobody wants to fund a trial for a treatment that can't be patented).

He was afraid we were wasting precious time, and we'd return worse off. When I pushed further and asked if he thought I could have 30 days to see if this alternative approach would have an effect, he begrudgingly said 30 days was ok, but not longer. Then he said if I didn't do anything, I would be dead within a year. Well that got my attention...

The fear was palpable. Clearly, I needed to do some serious soul-searching and make a decision quickly.

That afternoon, we met with Dr. B. for the 2nd surgical consult. She had a very different approach to my situation, and it didn't jive with me. She was clearly very intelligent, but she wasn't warm or genuine. I'm the kind of patient who really needs to feel cared for by my doctor.

When she first entered the room, she shook my hand firmly and asked how I had been sleeping. I responded, "Well, I was just told I have an aggressive cancer, so yeah, I haven't been getting a ton of restful sleep." Without knowing anything about me, she said she'd write me a prescription for Ambien.

Then she said, "I'm sure you're anxious, too, so I'll get you some Xanax." I was shocked at how quickly she was willing to put me on addictive medications. I politely refused and told her I'd prefer to work through it naturally.

She was incredibly thorough, walking us through a thick packet describing my diagnosis and what she planned to do, taking a pen and aggressively crossing out options that she didn't feel were right for me. For instance, she felt that there were some potential trouble spots (a shadow on my left breast, micro-calcifications on my right), and thus, she said I didn't qualify for a lumpectomy. She scratched a big red X across it with her pen, and then circled the 'bilateral mastectomy' option and said it was my only choice.

She wanted to get me into surgery right away, then wanted to do the same cocktail of 3 chemotherapy drugs that Dr. G. had mentioned. She told me to expect to have it rough for about 9 months to a year...

What was I in for? I have young children. I just couldn't imagine what my life would become, or how our little family was going to survive this.

She also wanted to order numerous tests "just to be sure". It was a long list of about 17 different types of diagnostic tests! This was very overwhelming and stressful. For some reason, I felt like I needed to cooperate, at least a little bit, so I agreed to do a blood draw to check my levels, to do an MRI to check the 'questionable' areas, and to do genetic testing, but said 'no for now' to the multitude of other tests.

I wasn't getting a good feeling from this surgeon. She didn't seem interested in getting to know me as the patient, as a HUMAN... she was making clinical decisions purely based on the pathology report. Didn't she want to know anything about me? Wasn't she interested in how *I* felt about moving forward on this path?

It's interesting how you sometimes feel the need to do

exactly what a doctor in a white coat tells you to do, especially when faced with something like cancer. You are extremely vulnerable and frightened, and it would be so easy to just say, "oh yes, of course. Whatever you think is best." I certainly felt that pressure.

However, I think doctors should encourage patients to take time to consider everything that they've been told; to discuss it with their spouse, perhaps, or their parents; to do research and learn about the pros and cons of all options before committing to something this big. It's a HUGE decision - these things that they were suggesting. And it just wasn't feeling...right.

THE CONSULT GETS COMPLICATED

"Always trust your gut. It knows what your head hasn't yet figured out." ~ **Author Unknown**

Dr. B. sent me downstairs to have my blood drawn, and to meet with the oncologist, Dr. J. Dr. J. was compassionate and patient. She calmly explained what she felt was the best approach, and she was willing to listen to my questions and my concerns. Yet in the end, her message was clear: the 'standard of care' indicated that I needed the triple cocktail of chemo.

She heard from Dr. B. that I wanted to try alternative treatments. She advised me against taking a month or two to see if that would have an effect before starting chemo, and instead said that I should consider doing it alongside the conventional treatment, perhaps to strengthen my body during the course of treatment. We discussed some of the potential side effects that I may experience, and she gave me a very large stack of material to take home with me.

As we were talking, my basic blood panel results came back,

and she found that my bilirubin was high. She pushed me to get an x-ray, a bone scan, and a CT scan to "see what's going on". However, I had been reading about the incredible amounts of radiation exposure involved with all of these tests. It gave me pause... was I creating more problems by having all of these diagnostic tests that were putting more of a toxic load on my body? My sensitive body that was trying so hard to heal itself??

"Like X-rays and PET scans, CT scans use ionizing radiation, which can damage DNA and **cause cancer**. Two other imaging technologies, MRI scans and ultrasound, do **not** use radiation. Studies published in 2007 and 2009 by teams from Columbia University and the NCI predicted that up to 2 percent of future cancers — about 29,000 cases and 15,000 deaths annually — might be caused by CT scans. A 2011 report by the Institute of Medicine found that the two environmental factors most strongly associated with breast cancer were radiation exposure and the use of post-menopausal hormones."

Taken from a Washington Post article, found here:

www.washingtonpost.com/national/health-science/how-much-to-worry-about-the-radiation-from-ct-scans/2016/01/04/8dfb80cc-8a30-11e5-be39-0034b-b576eee_story.html?noredirect=on&utm_term=.de61c1c8beac

I decided to take a copy of the blood results with me and investigate a bit further. I told her I needed the week to make some decisions on how to move forward before I did any further testing, besides the MRI and blood tests.

I went home and looked up all of my blood test results from over the years. I learned that the normal range for bilirubin was 0.1 − 1.2 mg/dL, and my history showed that I bounced around that range. Today, my 'high' bilirubin result was 1.3 mg/dL, barely out of the normal range. It seemed to me that this wasn't alarmingly high, and perhaps it would drop back into normal range once I had a handle on my current situation.

I declined the further testing, and I'm happy to report my bilirubin level did indeed return to normal without any intervention.

This was a valuable lesson for me: we all need to be aware of what our *individual* normal range is. The numbers that are used in the medical field are created by taking 95 percent of values from the general population, but each of our bodies are different in so many ways, and it's important that we are armed with our specific healthy ranges. If your normal is always closer to the high end, then perhaps being just outside of that high end isn't as worrisome. The old me would have heard the doctor say my level on this one reading was high and I needed testing to see what's going on, and I would have said, "Well, of course! Let's check it out! I hope you don't find anything terrible." And then I would have felt relief when nothing was found and thought that doctor was amazing. "Phew! Thank goodness it was a false alarm! I'm so glad you caught that before it became a problem!"

But instead, I didn't let one number that was barely outside of the assigned normal range to cause me to panic. The "wait and see" approach was key for me. Support your body in healing itself, as it's created to do, and it can do amazing things. The body wants to be in balance, so get out of its way and let it do its job. This was becoming my new motto.

CHOOSING A PATH

"You either get bitter or you get better. It's that simple. You either take what has been dealt to you and allow it to make you a better person, or you allow it to tear you down. The choice does not belong to fate, it belongs to you."
~ Josh Shipp

My Cancer Thriver friend and I had a long phone conversation after my Monday consults. She didn't feel that chemo was the right path for her, so after recovering from her double mastectomy, she went to the Hippocrates Health Institute. She learned about valuable lifestyle changes that would help her body remain cancer-free. She inspired me to make wheatgrass shots a daily part of my life. I also made sure to drink at least one fresh green juice every day.

www.hippocratesinst.org/comprehensive-cancer-wellness-program

It was an intriguing proposition, healing cancer naturally

without harmful drugs or radiation - but I needed more information to ease my mind. I've seen how chemo can destroy a person's immune system, and the side effects can be truly horrifying. There's the nausea, vomiting, and hair loss, but those are temporary (though still not welcome). More daunting was what they call 'long effects', such as heart problems or lung damage from chemo or radiation to the chest, hypertension that can cause organ damage, hearing loss, permanent neuropathy, hormone system problems, osteoporosis or rheumatologic problems, issues with your teeth or vision, cognitive impairment, and long-term digestion issues, not to mention that these treatments can cause OTHER cancers called Secondary Cancers! Wait, *what?!?* Yes, most chemotherapy drugs are known carcinogens. Well, that ain't good...

And how would my body be strong enough to bounce back after such an assault?? How would it be able to defend itself against future cancers if my immunity is compromised? It's such a daunting road... but NOT doing any treatments was clearly not an option. This was an aggressive cancer, and I felt the need to do something, and soon.

So we reached out to the filmmaker of the documentary *Cancer Can Be Killed* that my friend had mentioned.

Much to our surprise, he agreed to a phone conversation, and we immediately sat down with our note pads. He was open and honest about his experiences. He said his wife is still doing well, but if she ever needed treatment again, he would go to Marinus am Stein in Germany. His research for a follow-up documentary had led him to this small klinik in Bavaria, tucked in amongst the magnificence of the Alps.

We had already been researching Infusio in Germany and Sanoviv in Mexico with mixed results. So now we added Marinus to our list of possibilities.

TALKING TO THE KIDS

JUNE 26, 2018

"Today I refuse to stress myself out about things I cannot control or change." ~ **Author Unknown**

Tuesday, June 26th was another full day.

On the previous Sunday, I was able to sit down with a friend who had gone through a difficult stem cell procedure for a different illness a few years prior. She was also a mom of young children, and I had asked her how her kids took the news, and how they handled her illness. I was grateful to talk to someone who had survived a difficult period of her life and was now thriving, and I was so happy to hear that her children had handled the whole ordeal very well.

West and I didn't completely see eye-to-eye on whether to tell the kids about my diagnosis at first. I know that he wanted to protect them from the harsh reality of cancer, at least until it couldn't be hidden anymore (if I lost my hair, for instance), but I've always believed in total honesty and didn't feel right hiding anything from them. It had already weighed on me heavily in the handful of days since the call. I felt like I was hiding something really BIG, and they were picking up on my energy and asking questions.

My friend gave me excellent advice about how children are resilient (which is true), and how they can often handle more than we think (also true). After this talk, I felt in my heart that we should be upfront with the kids, in an age appropriate manner, so we could move forward as a team. However, West and I needed to be on the same page.

My good friend who was also healing from cancer told me about this amazing place called Wellness House in Hinsdale. https://wellnesshouse.org/

They offer tons of programs and services to cancer patients and survivors, completely free of charge. They happened to be offering a seminar that day called "Talking to Kids About Cancer", so I signed up, and we went to see what kind of helpful information we could gather.

This is where we first met Carly. She has been a Godsend, especially for our daughter (more about Carly and Wellness House later). Carly was leading the seminar, and we knew in an instant that she was special. She was kind and compassionate, but knew her stuff. We left 2 hours later knowing that we needed to have the conversation with the kids so we could all move forward together on a united front.

We sat them down around the kitchen table that evening. I started out by saying "Mommy is sick", but immediately it felt like I wasn't giving them the whole truth. At West's encouragement, I said, "I have cancer. But we are already making plans to kick this thing to the curb!"

We discussed how things might be a little different around the house. Mommy might be tired and not able to do some of the usual things, and they may need to help out a little more, but basically life would go on. Addison exclaimed, "We're gonna kick cancer's butt!!" And with that, I knew everything was going to be ok.

I still can't believe how well they rolled with it. No tears, not even much fear – hallelujah! Addison said she would grow her hair super long so we could make a wig out of it, since I'd always wanted curly hair (my heart melted). Hopefully, it wouldn't come to that. We shared that we were considering going to Europe for some holistic treatments that wouldn't make me feel sick, and they were all for it. They had a few more basic questions, and then asked if they could be excused to go play.

I found that using the word CANCER repeatedly and not shying away from it took some of the fear out of the word – it no longer had the same power to instill debilitating fear. Have you ever noticed when you dance around something and use words like "the C word" or "my illness", it feels like you are avoiding it or pretending it isn't really that serious? On the other hand, confronting it head on is empowering. I was taking the bull by the horns, and it gave me some control back over my life and my future.

It's funny. Right from the beginning, I fully accepted my diagnosis. I certainly wasn't happy about it, but I never had a moment of "why me?" or deep anger. I had cancer, and now I needed to take action.

It's like Eckhart Tolle says in *The Power of Now*, "Surrender (acceptance) is to accept the present moment unconditionally and without reservation. It is to relinquish inner resistance to what *is*. Inner resistance is to say 'no' to what *is*, through mental judgment and emotional negativity... Surrender is a purely inner phenomenon. It does not mean that on the outer level you cannot take action and change the situation.

For example, if you were stuck in the mud somewhere, you

wouldn't say: 'Okay, I resign myself to being stuck in the mud.' Resignation is not surrender. You don't need to accept an undesirable or unpleasant life situation. Nor do you need to deceive yourself and say that there is nothing wrong with being stuck in the mud. No. You recognize fully that you want to get out of it. You then narrow your attention down to the present moment without mentally labeling it in any way. This means that there is no judgment of the Now. Therefore, there is no resistance, no emotional negativity. You accept the 'is-ness' of this moment. Then you take action and do all that you can to get out of the mud. Such action I call positive action. It is far more effective than negative action, which arises out of anger, despair, or frustration. Until you achieve the desired result, you continue to practice surrender by refraining from labeling the Now."

This mindset has served me well on this journey.

LATER THAT EVENING...

"We cannot change the past, but the choices we
make today can change the future."
~ Christine Caine

My next goal for the day was to meet with Dr. W. - our final surgical consult, and the surgeon who had performed my friend's mastectomy. Thankfully, he had been able to sneak us in last minute at the end of the day. My awesome brother was willing to drop all of his plans and come to our rescue, driving the kids to various events and feeding them dinner (I'd be lost without my family and friends!).

Dr. W. was a wise, soft-spoken man. He'd been doing breast surgery for 25 years and had a quiet confidence about him (a welcome trait in a surgeon). After our consultation, we knew that he would be our guy, if we did indeed decide to go down this path. He had the experience and the knowledge, but he was also respectful of my wishes and how I wanted to heal my body.

I truly appreciated that, and knew that any doctor on my team had to be OK with my own choices about my care.

Instead of starting with surgery, he suggested starting with chemotherapy, so we'd have the tumor as a gauge. This would allow us to see if the approach was having an effect. This piece made a lot of sense to me – if we removed the tumor right away and then hit me with chemo, we'd have no way of knowing if it was truly effecting my specific cancer (though the more I considered all of the options, the more I was getting clear signals that chemo wasn't right for me, at any point in my care).

Perhaps we needed to take a monitoring approach, rather than a "get this s&!# out of me now!!" approach. Yes, it is a natural reaction to want the damaged cells, the tumor, to be removed from your body ASAP – it's scary as hell – but the more I was learning, the more I knew that cutting out the tumor was only a temporary solution.

Cancer is a symptom of a systemic problem. My whole body is sick, not just my breast. That just happens to be where the tumor took hold, but there was a serious problem with my immune system that was likely stemming from other issues in my life – diet, lifestyle, contaminants, stress... the list of possible contributing factors is long.

"The majority of treatments for cancer are extremely toxic, which further exacerbates the problem. Many cancer recurrences are likely due to the initial treatment. On the other hand, when you view cancer as a metabolic disease, you can target and manage the disease without creating systemic toxicity."
www.articles.mercola.com/sites/articles/archive/2019/01/06/metabolic-disease.asp

You see, we all have cancer cells in our bodies, but typically the immune system is able to identify these injured cells and eliminate them before they ever become a problem or are even detected. But the immune system can get overwhelmed, espe-cially with the incredible onslaught of toxic contributors in our world today, and while it's busy dealing with other toxins in our body, the cancer is given a chance to proliferate (divide) and grow. My cancer had a proliferation rate of 70%, meaning it was growing incredibly fast.

I was beginning to see that I could make a significant impact by making some major changes in my life. Which gave me a sense of control in this crazy whirlwind of a week.

MY HEALTHY LIFE NEEDS AN OVERHAUL

"Every time you eat or drink you are either feeding disease or fighting it!" ~ **Author Unknown**

It had only been 5 days since that fateful call. I was starting to get a handle on the possibilities, and I was beginning to see that I would need to tackle this from several directions in order to heal my entire system.

I was already leading a healthy life, or so I thought. I had studied at the Institute for Integrative Nutrition and was a certified health coach. So how could I be sick with a life-threatening illness?? Had I missed something along the way? I ate well the majority of the time, I did yoga regularly, and I believed in self-care.

But even with all of that, I often didn't put myself at the top of the priority list (though I knew I should). There were so many obligations and things pulling me in different directions. I rarely said "no" to requests of my time, to events and outings, to new opportunities. I would need to address my chronic stress, as well as take a good look at my food choices.

And I started by removing things from my plate, literally and figuratively.

My husband, West, has been an amazing support on this journey. Soon after the diagnosis, West and I decided to become strict Vegans. I knew that every bite of food I put into my mouth would either support my healing or fuel my disease, and he said that he wanted to support me fully so I didn't feel alone.

I was shocked, as were many people who know him, that this meat-and-potatoes man was willing to make such a radical move! It was incredibly touching, and if I'm honest, his solidarity would prove to be essential to my success in so many ways.

This new way of eating meant no animal products of any kind (goodbye luscious butter, bone broth, and salmon!), and we took it even further – no processed foods, no refined grains, no caffeine, no alcohol, and no sugar of any kind. Refined sugars, artificial sugars, honey, maple syrup – they were all off limits as some research shows that cancer cells thrive on sugar. Even fresh fruit was off the table for the first 30 days. I was determined to do everything I could to help my body heal.

**Please note: I'm NOT saying sugar *CAUSES* cancer – though there is no question in my mind that it is over-consumed, it is addictive, and it is generally not good for our health. In my personal opinion, I believe that it is indeed a factor.

Yes, all of our cells consume glucose, but the mere fact that they inject you with radioactive glucose prior to a PET scan so only the cancer cells "light up" shows that what I've heard is pretty accurate – that cancer cells consume glucose at a rate of 10 to 1 compared to healthy cells. It is a highly debated topic, but my philosophy is: why take the chance of giving the cancer more fuel? Sugar is a problem to our health on so many fronts, so eliminating or highly reducing it could only support my health over all.

"Given that several cancers express the insulin growth factor family of receptors on its surface, it is biochemically plausible that reducing sugar intake and thereby reducing insulin and insulin growth factor levels could help improve cancer outcomes in cancers that gain survival/growth benefits through that signaling pathway."

"Sucrose and fructose overconsumption in mice greatly accelerates the onset and progression of breast tumors in three different mouse or human breast tumor models through modulation of inflammatory pathways, independent of weight change or blood sugar" (Jiang Y, Cancer Research, 2016).

www.integrativeonc.org/news/research-blog/205-does-sugar-feed-cancer

I've read quite a bit about the Nobel Prize winning biochemist, Otto Warburg and his fascinating discoveries about cancer cells in the early 1900's. He found that cancer cells get their energy by fermenting glucose (aerobic glycolysis), rather than using oxygen respiration like healthy cells do.

> *"Cancer, above all other diseases, has countless secondary causes. But, even for cancer, there is only one prime cause. Summarized in a few words, the prime cause of cancer is the replacement of the respiration of oxygen in normal body cells by a fermentation of sugar."* ~ Otto Warburg

There isn't a lot of recent science to back up the claim that cancer cells devour glucose, but I believe it's returning to the forefront. I recently read a thought-provoking book called *Trip-*

ping Over the Truth written by Travis Christofferson, which provides detailed and significant evidence that we have been looking at cancer all wrong for a very long time. In the book, he discusses the world of cancer research, the figures influencing it, and the industry behind it. It's full of powerful insights about the triumphs and shortfalls behind the struggle against cancer. A must read if you have been touched by cancer.

A NEW PERSPECTIVE

"All that we are is the result of what we have thought. The mind is everything. What we think we become." ~ **Buddah**

As friends and family started to hear about my diagnosis, the calls, texts, and emails began to pour in. I found it difficult to respond to most of them – not only because my time was completely consumed with researching my options, but also because re-living the incredibly stressful details of my situation was taking an emotional toll on me. I simply couldn't bear to keep repeating this event over and over again.

I didn't have a lot of energy to respond, either. The past 7 days had been a whirlwind of consults, further testing, information gathering, and childcare scheduling, and I was exhausted from it all. I wasn't sleeping well because of the biopsy and the discomfort it created, on top of a mind that wouldn't stop swirling...

I asked my good friend, Jen, to create a private Facebook

group. It would allow me to share the details so everyone who was interested in following along could see it at one time. I know my friends are all busy and have lots to juggle in their own lives, so this provided an opportunity for them to get an update on their own time frame, without feeling obligated to have a lengthy phone call.

June 25, 2018 post:

"My sweet friend, Jennifo, created this amazing team of family and friends, and I couldn't be more grateful. It means so much to me to know that I'm not going to go through this alone, and I thank each of you for having my back! Love, prayers, positive healing vibes, friendship, and laughter are going to be the best medicine."

At first, Jen called it the "Army" made up of "warriors", brought together to "fight" the "battle" against cancer – all words typically used to describe a cancer journey. But those terms didn't feel right to me. While they were gearing me up for a war, they were also causing stress.

This wasn't going to be a single moment in time. This was going to be an on-going journey back to health. I would need to stay focused on healing every day.

And then I received this email from my insightful friend, Kevin:

"Leslie. Well, what a pain in the ass! And everywhere else. I am sorry to hear you have a new partner in life for a while: cancer. I say partner because while a friend of mine was managing her breast cancer, I listened to a lot of radio broadcasts about breast cancer...One of the interesting points of view was to stop discussing it as a battle. I found it crazy. But, the behavioral scientists said those terms release chemicals that inhibit healing. Weird, right? It puts you into battle mode, which is different from healing mode. I found it boggling. But, after reading many behavioral science books I can believe it."

His timing couldn't have been better, and his words resonated with me deeply. I know that combative thoughts and words put us into the "fight or flight" mode, releasing stress hormones such as cortisol and adrenaline into our system. These are very useful when you need to suddenly fight off a tiger, but if these hormones are coursing through our bodies constantly, it can be very damaging – especially when your body is trying desperately to heal cancer.

It made sense that focusing on a positive perspective would calm my system and support my healing. After all, this wasn't an accident that happened suddenly overnight. And this wasn't an invader from outer space. My body created this. Damaged cells bonded together to form a tumor – and my body would need to heal those cells, or perhaps eliminate the injured cells and create new healthy ones in their place.

So I decided that, for me, this wasn't going to be a battle to be won, or the fight of my lifetime. It was going to be a healing journey, full of love and friendship, full of support and nurturing, full of positive vibes and healthy thoughts.

I asked my support team to follow my lead - lean away from the combative language and thinking, and instead lean toward the healing language and thinking.

After all, on that fateful Thursday afternoon when I got the news, I accepted fully that I had cancer. Yes, there were moments over this journey when I felt intense fear of the unknown, but I didn't really experience denial or extreme grief. It was more a sense of, "Okay, this is the situation. Now what am I going to do about it?"

GATHERING INFORMATION

*"**I think it's brave** that you get up in the morning even if your soul is weary and your bones ache for a rest.*
***I think it's brave** that you keep on living even if you don't know how to anymore. **I think it's brave** that you push away the waves rolling in every day and you decide to fight yet again.*
I know there are days when you feel like giving up,
*but **I think it's brave** that you never do."*
~ Lana Rafaela

It was just over a week since the diagnosis, and I was still trying to figure out my path.

Through another amazing friend (I'll call her Gigi) I was able to get the name of a special Integrative Medicine doctor in Glenview who trained under Dr. Weil. She would understand my desire to boost my immune system and approach this in the most natural way, and I just knew that I needed to get in there soon.

When I called the appointment desk, they said her next

available appointment was in MARCH! I said, "I have an aggressive cancer and won't be able to wait 9 months to consult with her!" Yikes... Luckily, we have a family connection to Dr. Weil, and he generously stepped in and got me an appointment to see her at the end of that week. Thank you, Dr. Weil!

Unfortunately, she is out-of-pocket only, which I would find was quite common when diverting from the typical medical approach in the U.S.

West and I met with Dr. T and liked her very much. I also appreciated that she was in the same system as our surgeon of choice. She was not a cancer specialist, per se, but man, she knew her stuff! It was well worth the $450 to sit down with her and pick her brain. She was added to my team of doctors.

She had the paperwork all filled out to apply for my medical marijuana card and talked us through all of the steps. Man, they don't make it easy for you in Illinois. Even with a cancer diagnosis and a medical doctor signing off, it would take 90 days for them to process my card. I already knew how healing CBD is, and had recently been reading about the cancer healing properties of THC, but that would have to wait until the card arrived...

She also suggested a bunch of supplements and sent me to their store on-site with a list. We returned home with what seemed like dozens of bottles filled with pills for me to take daily. It was a little overwhelming, but I was ready to do whatever I could that wouldn't be damaging to my system.

The next day, I spent a lot of time reading through the plethora of information on the website, *Chris Beat Cancer*. Chris had been diagnosed 14 years earlier with colon cancer and had the tumor surgically removed. He then refused chemo and radiation, and instead radically changed his lifestyle. I would learn much from this man, and would depend on his guidance often as I moved forward. Check it out here:

www.chrisbeatcancer.com

What I love about Chris is how he not only focused on food, but also on many other elements of life that can affect our health and ultimately lead to disease, or potentially the healing of disease. I signed up for his *Square One* program and dove into healing daily.

I also watched the documentaries *What the Health* and *Forks Over Knives*, both offering valuable insights into the power of our choices. I was learning so much, and it was motivating me. I was feeling more and more like I could choose the non-toxic path and heal without the damaging effects of the conventional treatments being offered.

DO WHAT BRINGS YOU JOY

"When we sing our neurotransmitters connect in new and different ways, releasing endorphins that make us smarter, healthier, happier and more creative. And when we do this with other people, the effect is amplified." ~ **Tania De Jong**

July 1 was a big day. My sweet friend, Glenn, had invited my a cappella quartet, Route 66, to take part in a very special performance he was organizing, and we gladly agreed. What a wonderful opportunity to make music with some of my best friends!

But now my world was different, and I was dealing with a life-threatening disease that desperately needed my attention right now. Plus, my emotions had been rather raw for the previous 10 days... Could I really pull it together and do a live performance??

I went back and forth a bit, trying not to overwhelm myself. I'd already removed so many stressful things from my life in a short time. Would singing on stage at this moment of the journey be a positive experience, or would I simply be too distracted to focus on performing? Especially a cappella music, which offers no safety net from a band backing you up... it was daunting, for sure.

My amazing fellow singers/dear friends were nothing but supportive. They told me they completely understood if I needed to back out, considering everything I was dealing with at the moment, including possibly heading off to another country for treatments.

In the end, I decided that I needed to do the things that truly bring me JOY, and making music with my friends was one of those things.

I discovered that I was stronger than I imagined and was able to put aside everything that was going on in my life relating to the cancer and lose myself in the moment. It was a magical evening, and I'm so grateful to have had the opportunity to make music in the middle of the tornado happening in my life.

When we finished our last number and walked off stage into the wings, Glenn greeted me with one of his long and loving hugs. I fell apart and began sobbing. I had been holding in so many fears and emotions over the last week and half, and it was all coming out now. Then my 3 wonderful friends joined in on the giant group hug. We had pulled it off, and we had done it together.

This would turn out to be a resonating theme for my entire journey...

IS TESTING THE ANSWER?

JULY 2, 201

"*Learning how to say NO is essential because this practice is what gives us back our power.*"
~ Carley Schweet

I was off to get the MRI that Dr. B. had ordered. Dr. B. thought the test was necessary to gather more information on the micro-calcifications that had appeared in the diagnostic testing I'd done prior to June 21. There was also a small shadow on my left breast.

I'm not a fan of MRI's from my previous experiences...

I used to have debilitating migraine headaches. My PCP sent me to a neurologist who ordered an MRI of my brain (with and without contrast) and immediately put me on some pretty strong drugs. Of course, like all pharmaceuticals, these pills had some pretty bad side effects, one of which was SEVERE MIGRAINES!! And as fate would have it, that is what happened. The worst headache I've ever experienced – the kind that had me crawling under my covers to get out of the light, and putting in earplugs so my kids' laughing wasn't making my head explode. Not fun...

When I went for that very first MRI for the migraines, I had a panic attack shortly after being pushed into the tube and had to be removed quickly, which they explained was fairly common. They told me to get some anti-anxiety meds from my doc and then come back, which I did. I was able to successfully get through the MRI of my head because of the kind tech who put headphones on me and played music in my ears the entire time. I kept my eyes closed tightly and focused on choreographing a tap routine in my mind to the sounds of the machine happening around me. It was a wonderful distraction, and I was able to remain motionless for the entire test.

So when I went back for this MRI of my breasts, I was an old pro! It's still not fun, all of this testing – and there is always an element of stress involved, not to mention the time out of your schedule and the costs incurred. But the doctor told me I should do it, so who am I to say no....

Dr. B. called with the results, which were basically nonexistent. She could tell me nothing more than what we already knew.

My post to my group of supporters:

"The MRI was inconclusive. They want to run a bunch more tests.... Seems like Western medicine likes testing, cutting and heavy poison!! There must be a better way..."

Looking back, I wish I hadn't agreed to this test, or at the very least, been aware of the dangers of Gadolinium and only agreed to the MRI *without* contrast. There are now many people, including radiologists, who believe Gadolinium (the contrast medium that was injected into my bloodstream) can accumulate in tissues of the body, especially in the brain, causing damage *www.itnonline.com/article/debate-over-gadolinium-mri-contrast-toxicity*

The truth is, most of these tests and scans that they want to put me through expose me to harmful radiation and dyes, and will only make it more difficult for my body to heal itself. They tell me that it is "minimal" or "not enough to do harm", but the truth is it's cumulative over a lifetime. Each exposure is added on top of the ones before, and if you have a sensitive system like I do, you may be setting yourself up for trouble in the future.

I had been getting yearly mammograms for over a decade because of a benign breast tumor I'd had removed when I was 20 – could the cumulative radiation have been a contributing factor in my invasive cancer?? Could the ridiculous compression used in those mammograms have played a part? Nobody could give me definitive answers...

The only definitive information she had for us after the MRI was the size of the tumor – it measured 3.6 cm on the diagnostic mammogram that was taken on June 12, but now it was showing the tumor size was 3.2 cm. Could our diet changes be having an impact??

IS PATIENCE A VIRTUE?

JULY 3, 2018

"Patience is a form of wisdom. It demonstrates that we understand and accept the fact that sometimes things must unfold in their own time."
~ Jon Kabat-Zinn

At this point, we were seriously considering going to either Germany or Mexico for alternative treatments. And we wanted to be prepared to head off as a family at a moment's notice, if need be. Which meant we would all need valid passports, including the kids!

We did a little research, and discovered that adult passports are valid for 10 years, but the kids' passports were only valid for 5 years, so we needed to get them updated. We learned that you can get expedited passports if you apply in person, so we packed up the kids and headed downtown!

We made an event out of it, spending the entire day downtown together: First getting expedited passports; then getting fresh juice from Fruve on the south side (walking distance from the passport office); then we were actually able to eat lunch at a restaurant and stick to our Vegan Alkaline diet (thanks to the amazing True Food Kitchen and how accommodating they were); then I had a voiceover session while West and the kids played at Maggie Daley Park!

Yes, I was still working as a voiceover actor while trying to sort this cancer stuff out. I decided that the distraction of working would be good on some level (I love what I do, after all), as long as I didn't get too overwhelmed with the scheduling of the bookings. It did indeed make me feel, at least for an hour, that I was still living a normal life...

We were considering several places outside of the U.S. that offered alternative treatments. There was the clinic in Germany that was mentioned in the documentary *Cancer Can Be Killed*, but they weren't responding to our inquiry, which didn't instill confidence in us...

There was another 'med spa' in Baja, Mexico that sounded appealing because of the location by the ocean, and I loved their focus on healthy organic food and mind/body work. However, we had a phone consult with the doctor and he boldly told us he had never seen a tumor from triple negative breast cancer shrink from their treatments. The more we dug, the more we discovered that they were more of a 'health and wellness spa' and not focused solely on cancer treatments. It was sounding like this wasn't a good option for my particular situation.

Now our sights were set on Marinus am Stein in Brannenburg, Germany, the cancer clinic we learned about during the phone conversation with the filmmaker. He spoke highly of the doctor, and how he cared so much about his patients. It was a small family-run clinic that focused on holistic cancer treatments for many types of cancer.

We reached out to them and tried to arrange a phone

consult with Dr. Weber, but the time difference made it challenging (not to mention the language barrier). Patience was a difficult concept for me at this point in the journey. We sent over our reports and images and waited for a call, so we could make a plan to move forward. Time seemed to stand still...

THE HUG HEARD 'ROUND THE WORLD

"Your ability to stand up for your truth is a muscle, and the more you exercise it the stronger it gets."
~ Dan Pallotta

People were starting to ask me how I discovered the tumor. It's an interesting and confusing story, actually, and still a bit mind-boggling to me...

April 19, 2018

I had a full gynecological exam with Dr. Rock – no lumps or abnormalities detected during the physical breast exam, nor any pain under the pressure of his hands. All looked good! We agree that I was due for my annual mammogram screening, though we had no reason for concern. I wasn't in a huge hurry to get this painful and humiliating test done, so I put it off until June 4...

May 28, 2018 (less than 6 weeks after the exam)

While at a birthday party, I received an overly enthusiastic bear hug from a male friend, squeezing my chest into him with tremendous vigor. I felt a painful popping sensation in my right breast and exclaimed, "Oh my gosh, I think you just exploded my boob! Seriously, it feels like you popped my breast!" From that moment on, I had a 2-inch mass that could easily be felt with my fingers and was incredibly tender to the touch.

*Side note: Since this journey began, I've heard several people mention 'trauma-induced' cell changes... hmmm... I recalled that the tumor removed when I was 20 was also discovered after a swift elbow to my breast during a dance rehearsal. Coincidence??

The afore-mentioned mammogram screening: June 4, 2018

I went to Lutheran General Breast Center for my standard yearly mammogram. I undressed and got into the little paper gown and was led into the imaging room. The mammogram tech asked if there were any changes since my last screening – at first I said no, since I had gotten a clean bill of health from Dr. Rock on April 19. But then I off-handedly mentioned the crazy hug with a slight chuckle, and told her about the pain and thickness in that area. At this point, the tech refused to do the screening, stating that 'thickness' is one of the 12 signs of breast cancer. She said that I would need to call my doctor and get an order for a surgical consult and a diagnostic mammogram and ultrasound.

Thankfully, Dr. Rock – being supportive and awesome, as always – immediately called in the order. Much to my surprise, Lutheran General couldn't get me on their schedule for another week...

June 12, 2018

It was the day of the bilateral diagnostic mammogram and ultrasound, so I drove myself to Lutheran General.

It was a terrible experience – not only because of the fear that you feel when your mind is creating the absolute worst case scenario, but because of the unbearable pain that the mammo-gram caused.

Any woman reading this can understand the general pain and discomfort of a standard mammogram. But now imagine that same 42 pounds of pressure on a painful cancerous and invasive tumor!! The pain sent me to my knees in tears... She gave me a few minutes to pull myself together, and then we continued to get images from every angle. In fact, the first set of images they took weren't clear enough, so a half hour later, they brought me to another room to take more detailed images with a larger machine. More pain...

Then I was led into a separate room for the ultrasound. This was a BREEZE compared to the mammogram! Ultrasounds are not invasive nor painful - maybe just a little cold from the gel, though more places are incorporating a gel warmer, and that's a wonderful thing!

I waited to meet with the radiologist for the results. He was young, and I didn't care for the energy that he gave off, but he was the doctor who was assigned to talk to me, so I didn't even consider questioning it.

He said that I had a mass in my right breast measuring 3.6 cm, and we would need to do a biopsy to see if it was malignant (mammograms, ultrasounds and MRIs can't tell if a mass is cancerous – only the pathology from a biopsy can offer definitive answers). They scheduled the biopsy for a week later.

**Side note: some believe that compressing a cancerous tumor may cause trouble...

"Mammography can rupture tumors and spread malignant cells: Mammography involves compressing the breasts between two plates in order to spread out the breast tissue for imaging. Today's mammogram equip-ment applies 42 pounds of pressure to the breasts. Not surprisingly, this can cause significant pain. However, there is also a serious health risk associated with the compression applied to the breasts. Only 22 pounds of pressure is needed to rupture the encapsulation of a cancerous tumor. The amount of pressure involved in a mammography procedure therefore has the potential to rupture existing tumors and spread malignant cells into the bloodstream."

www.kresserinstitute.com/the-downside-of-mammograms

June 18, 2018

My husband drove me to Lutheran General for the biopsy. We waited for what seemed like an eternity. Once they finally took me in, and I was in my paper gown, I waited for someone to take me into the procedure room. The same radiologist from my previous visit entered the room. Could this really be the doctor who was going to perform my biopsy? I didn't have a good feeling... but I followed him like an obedient patient.

On my right side was the young doctor ready to do the surgical biopsy, and on my left side, was the ultrasound tech guiding the doctor with images. He made an incision in my breast, inserted the tool, and began to dig around, taking many samples. I was numbed from the pain, but it was incredibly uncomfortable.

It seemed like it was going on forever with him digging around in there, and then the tech said to him, "you need to go towards her feet – you're going towards her head. NO! Towards her feet!!" At this point, I had a really bad feeling.

I was already in a lot of pain from the procedure while getting dressed. They gave me an ice pack to help with the pain, and a 'goodie bag' containing pens and nail files with pink ribbons on them...

I headed home to discover that I was bruised significantly, and a large hematoma was forming under the incision. It only took 24 hours before the entire right side of my body was green and purple from the trauma. It was incredibly painful, and I had trouble sleeping for many weeks. The painful hematoma remained for months following the biopsy.

In hindsight, I should have trusted my instincts and asked for a different doctor. We all have the right to speak up when something doesn't feel right. I have learned so much from this journey.

*Side note: some believe that biopsies may spread cancer cells. Be aware of the risks and make the decision that is right for you.

https://www.ncbi.nlm.nih.gov/pmc/articlesPMC4015162/

GETTING CLOSER TO A PLAN

JULY 4, 2018

"Because the biological mechanisms that affect our health and well-being are so dynamic, when people change their diet and lifestyle, they usually feel so much better, so quickly, it reframes the reason for changing from fear of dying to joy of living. Joy of living is sustainable: fear of dying is not."
~ Dean Ornish

West's post to the new private Facebook page:

"Hello Everyone - This is a momentous occasion....I am making my first post on Facebook in my entire life. I apologize if I break some Facebook rules, but I am learning as I go!

If you don't want the details, you can skip down a few paragraphs and find the GENERAL PLAN section.

Here is a (not-so) quick update on what is going on in the world of "Kick Cancer's Butt!!" (Addison Robbins, 2018)

This week, as Leslie mentioned, she had an MRI. As she said, the MRI came back inconclusive for the micro-calcifications in the right breast (it is weird writing that word in public). However, we believe there was actually some good news in the report that our doctors don't recognize.

The mass was originally measured at 3.6 cm 2 weeks ago. The MRI came back and said it was now 3.2 cm, which was sort of perplexing to the doctor who gave us the update. She was surprised it was only that big, because the mammography, ultrasound, and her physical examination had pegged it to be much bigger.

My interpretation is that it's from all of the friggin' vegetables we have been eating. And yes, Mom & Dad, I am even eating KALE! Much to my chagrin, I do believe we are onto something here.

We continue to look into places to go and get non-toxic treatments. As of right now, we are focused on a German facility outside of Munich called Marinus am Stein. We are planning on speaking to them tomorrow and hope to be headed there very shortly.

We are very lucky that those in the community of cancer survivors are open and willing to speak to us. Many people have offered up their time to talk to us about their journeys, including people who have no connection to us.

For example, we had a chance to talk on the phone to the creator of *Cancer Can Be Killed*, and he was so helpful at putting our minds at ease about what we want to do. It continues to be an up and down ride, but things continue to trend upward.

GENERAL PLAN

This week: Finalize our plans to go to Germany (continue to be vegans)

Next week: Either get on a plane to Germany or prep for our departure (continue to be vegans)

Week of 7/16: We will be in Germany (continue to be vegans)

Week of 7/23: We will be in Germany (continue to be vegans)

Anyone seeing a trend here?!!!!!

We know that you are all thinking about us, and we very much appreciate it!! I will try to be better about updating everyone, but until now we really have had more questions than answers.

I hope you all have a great 4th of July!! Let's "Kick Cancer's Butt!!"

TOUGH KID-RELATED DECISIONS

JULY 4 – CONTINUED

"She made a promise to herself to hold her own well-being sacred." ~ **Author Unknown**

We had attempted to reach the doctor at Marinus am Stein in Germany (Dr. Weber) several times that day, to no avail. We needed to speak with him directly to discuss their program and his approach so we could make a final decision on how to proceed, but the time difference between Chicago and Bavaria made it quite difficult to catch him at the Klinik. We would try again tomorrow, and we'd set our alarm to wake up at 5 am to hopefully catch him before he headed home for the day at 2 pm Germany time.

I was getting quite anxious about doing SOMETHING, since I was keenly aware that the tumor was highly aggressive and proliferating at a high speed. Though I was more and more confident that I didn't want to jump into chemo, radiation, and surgery immediately as suggested by all of the western doctors, I knew that I needed to jump into some sort of treatment to get this thing under control, and FAST.

After all, it had already been 5 weeks since the appearance of the large and painful mass. I had changed my diet radically and attempted to reduce my stress, but it simply didn't feel like I was doing enough considering the severity of this invasive cancer.

I was feeling quite sure that a holistic cancer program in Germany was the right next step, but it was a huge commitment in so many ways. Not just the huge financial burden (it would be completely out of pocket – sadly, our healthcare system doesn't cover much in the way of alternative approaches), but also the scheduling of it. Was it smart to take the children along? At first impulse, it felt like the right move – to head to Europe as a family. It would be reassuring to have the love and support around me during this incredibly scary time.

I was also fighting demons in my mind... The pain in my breast notwithstanding, I surprisingly felt pretty healthy at the moment. But from the stories I was hearing of cancer patients who experienced a rapid decline, I was aware that my health could deteriorate at any moment. If these natural approaches didn't do what we hoped, and things took a turn for the worse, perhaps this would be our final family trip. The reality was difficult to process.

The more I thought about it the more I realized that stress was a big part of why this cancer was able to take hold in my body. I could feel the tumor 'engage' or pulse and ache whenever I would feel waves of stress. It sounds crazy because most breast cancer doesn't "hurt" – but mine did. And I knew it was my body speaking to me, telling me that I needed to be aware of my emotions and how they were affecting me... and the cancer.

Once I slowed down and got really honest with myself, I

knew that I'd be constantly worried about the kids if they came along, concerned about entertaining them, and how to feed them. I had been their main caretaker for the majority of their lives while West was traveling as a consultant, and it had taken a toll on me. I also knew that I needed to clear away many of my obligations and responsibilities, so I could truly focus on HEALING.

Perhaps we'd be smart to arrange for someone to stay home with them, so they could go to their summer camps and hang with their friends. And perhaps it was necessary for me to focus on taking care of myself, first and foremost...

SUPPORT IS EVERYTHING

"Anything is possible when you have the right people there to support you." ~ **Misty Copeland**

The power of the love and support from those on my 'team' cannot be overstated. It truly carried me through and helped me focus on staying strong and positive during this journey.

Early on, a dear friend of mine shared something she'd learned, and it rang true for me. She wanted to help somehow, and had chatted with another friend of hers who had also dealt with breast cancer.

Her friend told her that well-meaning people often say, "What can I do to help?" or "Let me know what I can do." I, too, have made this statement to friends going through tough times. Of course, the intentions are all loving and good, but she pointed out that this puts the burden on the person dealing with the disease or the loss of a loved one to come up with something you can do for them, or a time for you to do it.

It is all very much appreciated, but she was right – when

you lose a parent or receive a devastating diagnosis, you struggle to get through the day. Just showering and making dinner are tough at times. You are completely drained from the roller coaster of emotions, and it's tough to think straight.

So even though the person in need likely longs for the care and support, it is perhaps better to be very specific, if possible. State what you're willing to do for your friend going through the rough time. Make suggestions with specific dates when you're available to perhaps drop off a meal for the family or take the kids off their hands for the day.

This is exactly what my friend did – she made the initial offer to take the kids downtown for an overnight adventure and suggested several dates that could work. At first, it was too much for me to even consider or to schedule. We were in the thick of things, trying to determine our path, and were perhaps heading off to Europe with the kids at any moment. But I knew from her very sincere message that I could reach out to her at any point along the journey and take her up on her kind offer. And eventually, that's just what I did.

CARE PACKAGES THAT SUPPORT HEALING

"The struggle ends when gratitude begins."
~ **Neil Donald Walsh**

The care packages began pouring in, and it was both touching and humbling. People who loved me didn't hesitate for a moment to show me that they cared and would do anything to help. I could feel the love and it was keeping me strong. In the midst of this crazy cancer journey, I was feeling incredibly blessed!

If someone close to you is dealing with a health crisis, perhaps forgo the 'comfort food' and instead give them something that supports their health and healing. I know it seems supportive to send cupcakes, cookies, and all sorts of treats, but what they truly need now is something to *strengthen* them.

Maybe you could consider one of these thoughtful gifts that I received that was so meaningful on my journey:

- A beautiful teacup (green tea made from organic tea leaves is full of EGCG, a powerful antioxidant)
- Whole leaf tea from Real Tea Company (*www.rareteacompany.com*)
- Healing essential oils from doTERRA (some research shows that certain essential oils may be powerful tools when dealing with cancer: (*www.thetruthaboutcancer.com/essential-oils-for-cancer*)
- CD of Guided Mediation by Louise Hay called "Cancer - Discovering Your Healing Power"
- Healing stones and crystals (*www.goop.com/wellness/spirituality/the-8-essential-crystals*)
- Seaweed Bath Co detox soap (*www.seaweedbathco.com/products/detox-cellulite-soap*)
- Dried lavender for my kitchen and lavender satchels for the laundry
- Wool dryer balls (*www.amazon.com/Wool-Dryer-Balls-Pack-Organic*)
- Handmade knitted scarves
- Rejuvenating Rub, Lotion Bar, and Lip Balm from Moon Valley Organics (*www.moonvalleyorganics.com*)
- A purple DYLN water bottle that turns tap water into alkaline water (we were told that cancer cells thrive in an acidic environment, so we attempted to make my body alkaline. I have since learned that the cancer cells themselves create the acidic environment and drinking alkaline water won't

have a significant effect, but at the time, it was a positive step)

- The Essential Alkaline Diet Cookbook (West and I were very focused on alkaline foods for the first 30 days – combine that with our other long list of dietary restrictions and it became very difficult to maintain when you limit so many vegetables as well)

- Meaningful tokens such as necklaces, bracelets, socks with inspirational messages, healthy veggie-focused meals, empowering books on healing cancer and anti-cancer cookbooks, crystal angels, beautiful bouquets of flowers – all to remind me that I wasn't alone

YOGA TO THE RESCUE

JULY 5, 2018

"The quieter you become, the more you are able to hear." ~ **Rumi**

Europeans have a healthy work/life balance – Dr. Weber worked from 8 am until 2 pm, Monday through Friday, and then headed home with his wife, who also worked at the Klinik. We could learn many things from the European approach to life.

We set the alarms to be sure we woke up at 5 am in hopes of catching Dr. Weber before he left the office. I didn't *need* to set an alarm, as it turned out, since I hadn't been able to quiet my mind enough to actually fall into a deep sleep. With fingers crossed, we cleared our weary eyes and made the call again. This time, we got through to Daniela at the front desk. She said Dr. Weber was busy with patients, but she'd try to have him call us in the next hour.

We waited...and waited...and waited. By 7 am, I was beginning to lose my mind (lack of sleep certainly wasn't helping me think clearly). I tried doing some restorative yoga to help calm myself, but as I laid my body on the floor and swung my legs up the wall, I began sobbing uncontrollably. It was all becoming too much.

West stroked my hair and tried desperately to soothe my fragile nerves. I was thankful I wasn't alone, but also embarrassed that I couldn't control the sobs. I think I'd been holding in so many emotions for weeks and I simply couldn't contain it any longer. I was feeling so helpless and lost, without any clear direction.

It was now long after 2 pm in Germany, and we wouldn't likely be hearing from Dr. Weber that day. I finally got myself up off of the floor, still sobbing fiercely, and got dressed. I then decided to head to Yoga By Degrees for an 8:30 am class. Perhaps that would clear my head.

I walked up to the front desk and plopped my purple yoga mat on the counter. I gave my name to the kind teacher behind the computer, and as she checked me in for class, I thought it might be wise to let her know that my emotions were raw, and I might 'do my own thing' at times. After all, they often say that showing up to your mat and spending the entire hour in Child's Pose is still yoga at its essence... As I started to speak, the tears started to bubble up again.

She asked what was wrong, with sincere concern in her voice. I was barely able to mutter, "I was recently diagnosed with breast cancer," before the sobs burst out. I was falling apart, not able to control the fear inside of me. She rushed around the counter to console me with a hug and said, "You do whatever you need and whatever feels right. This is a safe space." Pamela became one of my all time favorite teachers.

TIMING IS EVERYTHING

"It takes courage to keep walking when the path is obscured by confusion.
Trust. Believe. And just keep walking. The way will be revealed" ~ **Sue Krebs**

Yoga was just what I needed to clear out the fear of the unknown after a long morning of waiting for the phone to ring. And Pamela was just the *teacher* I needed at that moment. I still attend her classes any chance I get. I so appreciate her gentle and supportive energy, and I always leave class feeling more centered than when I arrived.

When I got back to my car after class, I saw that a text had come in from West. Dr. Weber had stayed late that day to tend to his patients and had returned our call about 10 minutes into my yoga class. Timing is everything, as it turns out. But I still believe that the yoga class was a good choice for my mental health.

Thankfully, West was able to speak with Dr. Weber directly

and discuss all of our questions. He had gotten a really good feeling about Klinik Marinus am Stein and what they offer to cancer patients, but he especially liked Dr. Weber! He could tell that he was a genuine, kind-hearted man. West was convinced that this was indeed the place for us, and I trusted my husband's intuition.

Now that we'd found the treatment path that was right for me, I was anxious to get started as soon as possible! West and I agreed there was no time to waste. So we packed our bags, arranged for childcare, and were on a plane for Munich two days later.

We would fly out of Chicago on Saturday afternoon, the 7th of July, and arrive in Munich late Sunday morning. Marinus would arrange to have a car service meet us at the airport and take us to our new home for the next 3 weeks. I was a bit nervous, not knowing exactly what to expect, but I was comforted knowing that West would be by my side, and utterly thrilled to finally have a PLAN that felt right.

JULY 5 Facebook post to our "team":

"Update time: West and I have finally made a decision - we're heading to Germany!

Having a plan in place brings peace to my mind. We have been running non-stop for weeks, gathering information and talking to cancer survivors, and I'm so thrilled that we'll finally start taking some action!

Your continued love and support mean so much to us. It truly takes a village, especially when you get dealt an unexpected hand... we couldn't do this without all of you!"

HEADED TO THE KLINIK

"Surrender to what is. Let go of what was. Have faith in what will be." ~ **Sonia Ricotti**

West's mom flew in from Massachusetts, to stay with the kids. It was hard to imagine being away from them for 3 weeks, but it was clearly going to be much harder on me than it was on them! So many amazing people jumped in without hesitation to not only take the load off of Grandmom, but also to make sure the kids were distracted with lots of fun activities and not worrying about mom.

We had a direct flight from O'Hare to Munich, thank goodness, but it was still 9 hours in the air. Once we landed early the next morning, we made our way through customs and found our driver who would take us to our home for the next several weeks.

The clinic was about 90 minutes from the airport, and we enjoyed a beautiful tour of the countryside during the ride. Brannenburg is a small and quiet dairy town, and the clinic was on the outskirts, tucked in the middle of the Alps. I could tell immediately that it was a peaceful place and would be just the respite I needed.

As we pulled up to the quaint and very European-looking building that housed the clinic, I could already feel my stress fading away. We were far from typical daily life, and that was a good thing.

Daniela, the head nurse, greeted us and gave us a tour of the clinic before showing us to our little apartment next door. We unpacked and settled in a bit before heading to an early dinner with some of the other guests.

You could tell instantly that the people who come to Marinus are a unique lot, and the guests quickly bond over their shared experience. These people would become like family – a family of Cancer Thrivers who all wanted to approach this disease with a different attitude.

We had a chance to chat with several guests and were moved by how positive and supportive everyone was. We were particularly encouraged to hear their stories of healing!

One woman was diagnosed with breast cancer in May 2017, and it had metastasized to her bones. When she arrived at Marinus for her first visit, she couldn't walk without a walker due to 6 tumors on her spine and broken ribs from the cancer.

She stood in front of me now, talking about the hike around the mountains she had done that day. She was CANCER FREE, and back at Marinus for maintenance treatments to make sure the cancer never returned. I couldn't stop my tears from flowing... it was very inspiring to hear that you can actually turn stage 4 cancer around, without any chemo or radiation. My faith was getting stronger!

HEALTHY FOOD & YOGA

"Food is information, not just a source of energy or calories. It contains instructions that affect every biological function of your body."
~ Dr. Mark Hyman

Unfortunately, those running this program didn't seem to believe in the impact that nutrition and lifestyle can have on our health, which was disappointing, because that's what I'm all about.

I actually had to walk out of the dining room (politely excused myself) because the chocolate bars came out and were passed around to all of the patients.

It boggled my mind - why would they encourage cancer patients to eat overly processed garbage like this? Fried chicken wings were on the menu, and big steins of beer and glasses of wine were served at both lunch and dinner. But I had learned that alcohol was like throwing gasoline on a fire when it comes to cancer... it just didn't make sense.

Looking back, I can now appreciate that each person has to travel their own journey and do what is right for them, but this was my first day, and I expected a program that focused on holistic treatments to heal cancer would embrace the "let food be thy medicine" approach to health as well.

I had learned so much in a short time about the powerful effects that foods can have on cancer, both positive and negative - and I desperately wanted that to be a part of my "toolbox".

Thankfully, with West's help, we were able to stay 100% committed to our vegan, sugar-free, gluten-free, caffeine-free, alcohol-free diet (we were even FRUIT-FREE for the first 30 days).

The silver lining: the kitchen staff at Marinus was incredibly accommodating. Not only did they make us a special salad of corn, carrots and cucumbers (unfortunately with a very sugary dressing), but we found when we spoke up and asked for what we needed to stay true to our path, they were more than happy to order specific things for us, such as avocados, almonds and coconut milk!

It was a valuable lesson - we all have the right to ask for what we need, and if it's done in a respectful manner, most people are happy to oblige.

Another thing missing at the clinic was the yoga/meditation/mindfulness piece of healing, so I knew I had to take that element into my own hands. Luckily, I packed my purple yoga mat in my very large suitcase.

Marinus is surrounded by glorious mountains and has a beautiful lush green garden in the backyard, so I was able to plop down my mat outside and do a daily practice, accompanied by an awe-inspiring panoramic view!

It was nurturing to my soul, and I was so grateful. And I'm

happy to say it inspired others! It prompted many conversations about the power of yoga and how important it is to our healing to slow down and make time for ourselves. ❤

BEAUTIFUL DAY IN BRANNENBURG

JULY 9, 2018

"If it doesn't challenge you, it won't change you.
Growth happens in the uncomfortable spaces."
~ Author Unknown

I posted the following in the private Facebook group page, after my first full day at the clinic:

"Today was a beautiful day in Brannenburg, for more reasons than one...

It is a sunny day and about 78° - simply gorgeous! West and I took a long walk through the countryside admiring the cute Bavarian houses and amazing views. We've met such lovely people, both the guests and the staff.

We had a meeting with Dr. Weber this morning. We like him very much! He is kind, but also very passionate about what he does. He laid out the plan for us with all of the treatments for my specific cancer and gave us the supplements that I'll be taking daily. We talked to him about our vegan / alkaline / no sugar / no gluten diet, and he was supportive. He believes each patient should do whatever they need to do to get their mind in the right place.

On a similar note, we're happy to report that the kitchen at Marinus has been very accommodating, and has served us roasted vegetables or some sort of ratatouille or a salad for every meal! We even got to eat oatmeal with coconut milk this morning, and it was a deliciously special treat. ☺

I'm also delighted to learn that there is a bit of self-care included in the program - the doctor has scheduled me for 3 massages and 2 Reflexology treatments each week! In addition, I'm able to do my yoga DVDs and meditation daily in our cozy room.

Each day we meet more patients who share their amazing transformational experiences happening here, and it's so inspiring! We met a spunky outgoing man from Texas who had stage 4 lung and prostate cancer three years ago - he is now cancer free and is back for maintenance!

He told me how the Western docs said there was nothing else they could do for him and basically sent him home to die. He decided to come to Marinus and see if it might help. His entire family came to Europe with him, thinking this may be their last trip together. He now returns to Marinus with his lovely wife 3 times a year, and various family members still join him. He gets a full week of treatments, and then they tack on an additional week's vacation to a different European country (this time, they're headed to Italy!).

At dinner we learned that Carol, who was also stage 4 with metastasis to her liver, had an ultrasound today, and her liver tumors have DISAPPEARED after just 2 weeks of treatment!

Every single person here has made progress toward health, and it's so encouraging!

Now, on to the best news...

My day has consisted of:

- A Thymus shot in my a** (youch!)
- A large blood draw (5 vials!!)
- Ozone Therapy where they remove 50 ML of my blood, oxygenate it and then put it back into my body
- An IV infusion of selenium and folic acid
- Magnetic pulse therapy (I could feel it working! The tumor was MAD)
- Oxygen Therapy and BioMat (West will explain each treatment in detail in a separate post)
- Hyperthermia Therapy

AND

- an ultrasound- this is the exciting part...

My MRI, from last week, showed a potentially suspicious area in my left breast, and we were told to get an ultrasound to determine if it was something to worry about. The ultrasound today showed NOTHING abnormal in my left breast, and even more exciting, she checked my lymph nodes, spleen, gallbladder, liver and kidneys and they all were CLEAR!! YAY! What a load off my mind...

We also were amazed to hear that the tumor had shrunk even more since last week!! It started at 3.6 cm at diagnosis, then was 3.2 cm in the MRI and today measured 2.8 cm! We're more determined than ever to stick to this healthy diet and stay true to this path of healing – IT'S WORKING!!"

DETAILS & MORE DETAILS

"Reminders when healing: consistency counts; patience over speed; be gentle with yourself; it won't happen overnight; new habits equal a new life; there will be ups and downs; the seeds we plant will bloom." ~ **Yung Pueblo**

It was now time for me to focus solely on my healing and remove myself from the responsibility of keeping everyone updated back home. Thankfully, West was willing to take this on, and did a terrific job posting daily with details on our various events in Germany.

West's post to the Facebook private group page on July 10:

"We don't know who knows what, so here is a quick description of Leslie's diagnosis that we are addressing.

The cancer is a Grade 3, Stage IIB invasive ductile carcinoma. Here is what that means:

Grade 3 means it is an aggressive form of cancer that is multiplying rapidly. Stage IIB means that it is between 2 cm and 5 cm, it has not metastasized, and it is a triple negative cancer. Triple negative cancer means that it doesn't have Estrogen, Progesterone, or HER2/neu receptors - In essence that means it is not treatable through hormone therapy. Therefore, all conventional medicine doctors say you should treat this with chemotherapy and then cut it out through surgery. Today starts our journey to avoid the chemotherapy.

Day 1
        Guten Morgen-
        As we had heard from all of our new friends here, Day 1 was very busy. We first had breakfast - the staff has been very understanding and cooperative regarding our very restrictive diet. Then we did some paperwork, met with Dr. Weber who talked through the various treatments with us, and then it was off to start the healing process.
        The following is the list of treatments she was given on Day 1. I have tried to provide my best understanding of the "purpose" of each treatment. (I may have gotten a little geeky in some areas)

    • Thymus Peptide shot in the butt

The purpose of this treatment is aimed at strengthening the immune system and thus enhancing the defense reactions of the body. It also promotes the creation of antibodies against cancer-cells.

    • Blood draw for testing (5 vials for initial blood tests)

Multiple tests are performed on her blood to get the base

levels. This will help them determine if they ne[ ] course of action after next week's blood tests.

- Ozone Therapy IV drip (50 ml of blood oxygenated by adding O3, then reintroduced to her body)

Cancer does not like a highly oxygenated environment. This is aimed at letting it know it is not welcome here anymore.

- Selenium IV drip (essential trace mineral)

This is an antioxidant that focuses on eliminating free radicals that want to damage healthy cells. It is also working on prohibiting the growth of the cancer cells.

- Folic acid IV drip (and Vitamin B1, B6, and B12)

Folic acid is a key vitamin that is essential in the accurate reproduction of the cellular blueprint, as well as the production of red blood cells. It supports Vitamin B-12, which is essential in over 300 enzymatic reactions and is a key element to proper cellular system function.

- Met with Steffi (Head Nurse) to get the weekly schedule

- Magnetic field therapy (Frema-magnetic field) targeted at the tumor. They place an electrode just over the tumor and send magnetic pulses through the tumor. It is aimed at blocking the development of blood supply for tumor growth and also exacerbating the inherent instability in the genetic code. This has been shown to target cancer cells only. In addition, it strengthens the healthy cells around the cancer by raising the charge of the cells, which attracts more oxygen (cancer doesn't like oxygen) and clears out toxins. (She felt zingers during and after the treatment that made Dr. Weber happy - he said "dat is goot!")

- Lunch (Awesome Roasted Vegetables)

- Massage followed by rubbing alcohol rub-down

Get the blood circulating through the body and help general blood flow to keep things moving!

- Biomat pulsating magnetic fields and Oxygen

She lies on a bed of electrodes and is given oxygen through a nasal cannula. The goal here is to strengthen the rest of her body through enhancing blood vessels, improving blood circulation (especially microcirculation), and increasing the body's ability to absorb oxygen. In general, it increases the metabolism and optimizes the energy supply to the cells thereby increasing overall efficiency (we engineers love this) of the self-healing forces.

- Ultrasound (See below for more details)

Reviewed her Kidneys, Liver, Gall Bladder (she has gallstones, but no big deal), Spleen, Left Breast and Right Breast, and the tumor. As Leslie said, all other organs look normal! The only issue is the tumor.

- Hyperthermia

Focused radio waves on the affected region increases the temperature to a level where the cancer cannot survive (42°C / ~108°F). Pretty cool technology. She lies on a waterbed to keep her cool, while two terminals pass radio waves back and forth that, in essence, increase the temperature of denser material, such as a cancerous tumor.

- Dinner (delicious and very garlicky vegetables – garlic is shown to kill cancer cells)

We have been taking walks around the area. It is a very nice area with single lane roads, no sidewalks, amazing scenery and lots of nature. There is a stream with some mini waterfalls nearby that we like to go watch. We have also heard from other patients that there are some bigger waterfalls within walking distance as well as some castle ruins. I am looking forward to checking those out.

Leslie has met a friend that we visit daily - a young calf at one of the barns. They like to play together!

Details on the ultrasound of the tumor:

When Leslie first had her diagnostic mammogram, the largest dimension that was measured was 3.6 cm. If you recall on my last post, the MRI had shown the largest dimension to be 3.2 cm. Today, in the ultrasound, the largest dimension the doctor could measure was 2.8 cm. All of that was before we even started any of the treatments. We are feeling very optimistic about saying goodbye to this unwelcome guest.

In addition, she has been given several supplements that she has to take daily.

- Bee Pollen

Rich source of many vitamins and minerals, along with carbohydrates and proteins. By the way, it isn't honey and tastes like monkey ass, I am told.

- pH Balancing

Cancer thrives in an acidic environment. This can be brought on by the foods you eat (sugar, meat, etc.), stress that produces cortisol which is acidic, and many other things. Your body's natural state is alkaline; therefore, anything you can do to promote an alkaline environment is good for the body.

- Ortho Molar Pro

High Concentrations of vitamins and minerals in conjunction with a probiotic for gut health."

TO BRA OR NOT TO BRA?

"Focus on what you can change and let the rest go"
~ Author Unknown

A friend who I've known for many years responded to the detailed first post. She recommended that I avoid wearing a bra and keep moving and exercising as much as possible...stating that the body releases toxins through the skin – approximately 2 pounds daily. She said to wear loose fitting clothing and if you can, natural fibers. All excellent suggestions to help support my healing.

These were interesting points to consider. We were very focused on food, reducing my stress, and the power of alternative treatments, but I hadn't yet taken time to consider other factors.

Movement has always been a big part of my life, either on stage as a dancer or as a student of yoga. I knew how essential it was to keep moving each and every day, but hadn't truly considered how this could help my body heal from cancer. The walks every evening or bike rides and hikes in the countryside would become a priority.

The idea that constrictive clothing, such as a bra, could hinder my body from clearing out toxins hadn't really occurred to me, but now I was intrigued. I've always been more comfortable in loose fitting clothing that allowed easy movement, so at least I was on the right track there.

I did a little research on how bras could be troublesome. A lot of articles came up, but this one made a lot of sense to me:

www.goop.com/wellness/health/could-there-possibly-be-a-link-between-underwire-bras-and-breast-cancer

I appreciate how the doctor who wrote the article doesn't launch into fear tactics, but calmly discusses the research and then suggests that there could be logical connections between wearing a bra and lymphatic drainage, additional EMF exposure and even the temperature of the breast tissue. The doctor never states that bras *cause* cancer, but simply discussed how a bra might inhibit the natural functions of our amazing body. Food for thought, if you will.

I shared the article on my personal Facebook page to help spread awareness and provoke others to consider these views. Almost immediately, a comment was made, stating, "I promise you your bra and deodorant have nothing to do with getting breast cancer."

I was surprised that someone could make such a definitive statement. How could anyone say with certainty that these elements aren't in some way a factor? Even cancer researchers admit that cancer is confounding, and there is so much even they don't understand about its root cause.

In my opinion, it made sense to make whatever small (or large) changes I was able to make in order to help my body heal. Each of these pieces would hopefully add up to a stronger immune system that could heal the cancer, without needing to turn to poison in the form of chemotherapy or harmful radiation.

It was a no-brainer for me – I would ditch the bra whenever feasible (which, much to my mother's dismay, was most of the time) in support of my health.

It most certainly isn't just one factor that allows the cancer to take hold and grow out of control, and it most certainly wouldn't be one treatment or one change that would heal me. I needed an entire SHIFT in order to return to health. This was going to be a long and winding road...

DAY TWO AT MARINUS

JULY 10, 2018

"Maybe the hardest part of life is just having the courage to try." ~ **Rachel Hollis**

West's post to the Facebook private group page:

"Day 2 -

Our little apartment is great! We love it, but the beds are too hard for Leslie right now. She isn't sleeping well, but hopefully she will get used to it.

So far, she has been mostly pain free. She gets zingers in the tumor from time to time, which I would assume is a good thing.

Today's treatments and activities include:

- Breakfast (Oatmeal with Coconut Milk and some Vegetables)

We are seated with two women from Huntsville, AL, with Russian Accents. This is one sister's second trip here. The first time she left cancer free, but recently had a small tumor reappear. We discussed what and why we are eating the way we are. She was very intrigued because she says she is eating very healthfully and was surprised it came back. We talked about what we had learned, and we could see the wheels turning.

- Reflexology

The focus of this treatment is to bring about a feeling of wellbeing and help boost the immune system.

- Thymus Peptide shot in the butt for immune system support

- Mistletoe Extract Injection

Stimulation of the immune system - studies have shown that Mistletoe is an active cancer cell killer! Take that, you unwelcome guest!

- Magnetic field therapy (Frema-magnetic field) focused on the tumo

- Biomat pulsating magnetic fields and Oxygen

- Ozone Therapy IV drip (50 ml of blood removed, oxygenated by adding O3, then reintroduced to her body)

- Vitamin C IV drip

High dose IVC is an antioxidant that helps to eradicate free radicals and support the immune system. (I am going to get geeky here) In addition, recent studies show that it easily breaks down, generating hydrogen peroxide, a so-called reactive oxygen chemical that can damage tissue and DNA. Cancer cells are much less capable of removing the damaging hydrogen peroxide than normal cells thus killing the cancer cells.

- Artemisinin IV drip (comes from a common garden plant artemesia or wormwood)

It induces natural cell death in human cancer cells. Some studies show that it actually seeks out and destroys invaders like breast cancer cells. Geeky Information: Iron is used to help in the reproduction of cells and DNA. Cancer cells typically have much higher iron concentrations. They also have many more so-called transferrin receptors than normal cells have. Transferrin receptors are used to transfer iron into the cells. The treatment consists of two compounds called holotransferrin and artemisinin. The holotransferrin is used by cancer cells to help transfer even more iron into the cell therefore increasing the iron concentration of the cancer cells even more. Then, the artemisinin is introduced and combines with the iron in the cells and basically causes (in my mind) an explosion, destroying the cancer cell

- Lunch (Salad with a lemon citrus dressing and vegetables in a broth

- Bike Ride

We took a bike ride into the town today to get some money, shampoo, conditioner, and other toiletries. It was an easy ride and we enjoyed it

- Hyperthermia - High heat treatment focused on the tumor

- Dinner (Roasted Vegetables and some Vegan Soup

- Movie

(Devil Wears Prada)"

DAY THREE AT MARINUS

JULY 11, 2018

"I don't understand why asking people to eat a well-balanced vegetarian diet is considered drastic, while it is medically conservative to cut people open and put them on cholesterol lowering drugs for the rest of their lives." ~ **Dr. Dean Ornish**

West's post to the private Facebook group:

"Day 3 -

Today is a lighter day in terms of the treatments, which is probably good given that her arm is hurting today from the Mistletoe Injection yesterday.

- Urine Sample and Free Radical Test – We forgot she needed to do a urine sample yesterday morning, so she had to bring one to the lab today. While she was there, they pricked her finger to get a measurement of her Free Radicals. They really had to squeeze her finger hard in order to get enough

blood out for the test – she is very stingy that way
;). See Blood Work Results below for an update.

- Breakfast (Oatmeal with Coconut Milk and some
  Vegetables)

- Thymus Peptide shot for immune system support

- Blood Work Results

We got some more good news today. All of Leslie's blood
work tests came back in the normal ranges including thyroid
and red and white blood cell counts. Even the cancer marker
(CA 15-3) came back in the non-cancerous range (Leslie's level:
14; any number >30 indicates a tumor). The CEA, which is
the whole body marker (meaning the cancer has metastasized),
came back in the non-cancerous range as well.

Conversations with Dr. Weber brought to light the relia-
bility of the results - only 60% of the time does the test correlate
- we aren't sure why they bother doing the test. Her bilirubin
had also dropped down to well within the normal range – not
sure why it was high the week we left.

The only issue that she has is that her free radicals are high
(Leslie's level: 374; Normal range: 300). Again, Dr. Weber was
not too worried about it. They gave Leslie 3 options for how to
treat this issue: eating dark chocolate, having a footbath several
times a week, or taking 6 supplement tablets a day. Can anyone
guess which one we chose?!?! Yup, we chose the foot
bath!! Fooled you, we are serious about our alkaline diet and
cocoa is very acidic to the body!!

- Lunch (Salad, Quinoa with zucchini and mushrooms, yum!)

- Detox Foot Bath

- Massage followed by rubbing alcohol rub-down

- Magnetic field therapy (Frema-magnetic field) focused on the tumor

- Biomat pulsating magnetic fields and Oxygen

- Bike Ride

We rode up to the bottom of the Wendelstein Cog Railway, which takes people to the top of the mountain. It looks gorgeous, so we are kind of excited to go explore it. Probably next week, we will try to go up the mountain! As always, we had to stop by and see our friend 75 744 (the calf at the dairy farm). He was less playful today. We think he got in trouble with momma, because he wouldn't come out of his house.

- Hyperthermia - High heat treatment focused on the tumor

- Dinner (Indian Vegetable Rice dish)

We got to speak to the kids tonight and each of our moms and sisters. Then it was off to bed as we were exhausted."

DAY FOUR AT MARINUS

JULY 12, 2018

"Never let a bad situation bring out the worst in you. Be strong and choose to be positive."
~ Author Unknown

West's post to the private Facebook group:

"Day 4 -

There aren't any new treatments today, so it will be a relatively short post. However, I wanted to talk about Dr. Weber a little today. When I was researching this place, I read about how nice everyone was and how caring Dr. Weber was. I wanted to add some more color to that as we have had a few experiences here that are amazing!

When we first met with Dr. Weber that first day, he was so nice and affable. Once we understood his sarcastic humor, he is actually quite funny. Leslie says that he and I are having a "bromance" because we make each other laugh.

Despite Leslie's aversion to taking pills, Dr. Weber and I decided she should take the Free Radical pills, but use Bavarian

Beer to wash them down instead of water! ;) Haha – just kidding!

He is always very concerned that Leslie is happy and comfortable with any decisions that are made. He believes that your head needs to be behind your actions. He is like that awesome uncle who always makes you laugh and genuinely has your back.

One additional story I want to share about him that we heard from another patient who has been here before. A little aside about her (we'll call her T): She went home the first time breast cancer free, then went back to her normal life in every way – food, lifestyle, stress levels, etc. A couple of years later, the cancer came back and had spread to her bones. This time she has been here for 5 weeks already and is seeing some improvements; we are anxiously awaiting an update on her situation.

Sorry, I digressed.

It seems that Dr. Weber was partners in another Klinik about 12-15 years ago. Supposedly, it was quite success-ful. However, his partner seemed to be more interested in the money than in taking care of the patients. This is reportedly why they went their separate ways and he started Klinik Marinus am Stein.

We have found his generosity to be completely true, given the speed at which we wanted to get here. We made the deci-sion to come last Thursday and were on a plane on Satur-day. Prior to our arrival, they required us to only send a deposit of about 1/3 of the costs (all of the other places required you to pay in full upfront or they wouldn't start treatment).

So we quickly initiated the wire transfer from Chase and despite some snags with the bank (it is actually good they are so concerned about identity theft), the wire was submitted. Initially, the bank told us it would take 1-3 business days for the wire to arrive. We have been checking daily and in the last communication Chase changed their story to 3-5 business days because it is international. As of today (the 5th business day), the money still hasn't been sent to the Klinik, which is frustrating!!

On Tuesday, Petra (Dr. Weber's wife, who is also a doctor here) came to us to ask us where the money was. Her biggest concern was that it might have been hacked (another patient had this happen to them), not that it was late but that it was stolen! We offered to give them our credit card and she said not to worry - she knows it will arrive soon. I was completely floored by that conversation! We have had 4+ days of treatments, accommodations, and food, and they aren't worried about the money. I, on the other hand, am completely embarrassed and very angry with Chase right now."

DAY SIX AT MARINUS

JULY 14, 2018

"A good laugh and a long sleep are the two best cures for anything." ~ **Irish Proverb**

West's post to the private Facebook group:

"Day 6 –

Leslie had a rough night last night. She had a hard time sleeping, despite the new pillow that has allowed her to get some rest. Curse you Chase Bank!

Many of our friends left this morning to head back to the U.S. Every one of them had some very positive news upon leaving. Dr. Weber told one woman who was given 12 months to live by doctors at home, that she doesn't have to come back for 6 months because her body is responding so well to the treatments. Another guy who had prostate cancer was told by Dr. Weber he doesn't need to come back EVER!"

Friends reached out regarding the sleep challenges, offering some suggestions. One struggled with insomnia and suggested a cold & dark room, a warm bath before bed, deep breathing, and a heavy blanket. Another friend recommended using essential oils – lavender oil and lotion rubbed on your arms or used during a nice foot rub prior to bed.

Yep, all of those things help me sleep better on a typical night. We have blackout shades in all bedrooms at home and keep it quite cool; I often throw my legs up the wall and do some deep breathing; I have a diffuser next to my bed with lavender and peppermint essential oils that help relax me after a long day; I use a noise machine to block out the sound of the planes overhead or trucks on the nearby road; and I especially love a warm detox bath of Epsom salts, baking soda and lavender oil – unfortunately, we can barely stand up straight in our shower at Marinus... so no baths for us while in Germany. Keeping the room cool was impossible – it was July and there was no air conditioning at the Klinik (we did have a small fan, but that could only do so much). There also weren't shades on the windows, so darkness was a bit tricky once the sun came up.

Here are some more thoughts on getting a good night's sleep:

www.drweil.com/health-wellness/body-mind-spirit/sleep-issues/natural-sleep-aids-tips

DAY SEVEN AT MARINUS

JULY 15, 2018

"Unchangeable conditions are only 'unchangeable'
because you believe that they are."
~ Author Unknown

West's post:

"Day 7 -

Today was moving day! We had to move out of our cute little apartment and into the Klinik today. Leslie slept better, which makes her mood better.

We took a quick 15-minute ride to Lake Hawaii See this afternoon. It was really nice getting there (all downhill), not so much coming home!

Day 8 (July 16) -

Our first night in the new room went ok and we got some decent sleep. And now that we are in the Klinik itself, we can have laundry done! Yay for no more smelly clothes!

A new crop of patients arrived today. It is weird feeling like the elder statesmen! We look forward to hearing all of their stories. Leslie got to chatting with a woman today during one of her treatments. As it turns out she is from Holland! Leslie was so excited to use her Dutch again!

Leslie and I are on the same floor as Dr. Weber's office. We were hanging out in a lounging area as he started to walk by. He sees me and says, "You are Vegan!?" I was pretty astonished that he knew that about me, and that he was focused on me and not Leslie.

I said, "Yes, for 3 weeks now!" Leslie pipes in and says he has lost a lot of weight, too!

Dr. Weber says, "Really?!?! Maybe I turn Vegan!" I told him that he could still have his Bavarian Beer if he did. We all had a good laugh. He is such a genuinely funny and nice guy.

- Liver Pack

Our first new treatment in a while. The nurse shows up at the room at 11:00 am and rubs almond oil over her liver, then places a hot towel over it, a heating pack, and then another towel. She has to lie on her back for 45 minutes while the heat does its thing. The purpose is to help the liver detoxify itself."

DAY NINE AT MARINUS

JULY 17, 2018

"It's more important to understand the imbalances in your body's basic systems and restore balance, rather than name the disease and match the pill to the ill." ~ **Mark Hyman, MD**

West's post:
"Day 9 -
The second night was much better at the Klinik. She seems to have gotten more sleep, and her mood reflects it.

We got some surprising news today. We expected to have an ultrasound each week to see how the treatment is progressing. What we were told today by the nurse is that we won't have another ultrasound until the end of our visit. Darn...

We took an evening walk to go see 75 744. He seemed to be more interested in his dinner than playing with Leslie. The weather here is beautiful and the scenery continues to amaze us."

. . .

"Day 10 (July 18) -

We had a quick conversation with Dr. Weber today. He is always here, which definitely gives us comfort. We asked about her blood test results and he said everything looks great, but once again the markers only show up 60% of the time in confirmed breast cancer cases.

We asked how we would know if the protocol needs to be changed. As we had hoped, he said we should come find him and have an ultrasound tomorrow. So we are excitedly awaiting the ultrasound results.

Two things we are learning here is that the patients are a wealth of knowledge, and that you have to advocate for yourself. Many of the repeat patients have talked about different therapies, diets, or tests they have had done, and the advantages and disadvantages of them. It is amazing how many different options are out there, but it can be a little overwhelming.

Specifically, we keep hearing from other patients about 'this type of diet' or 'that type of diet' that seems to work for them or someone they know. However, my engineering brain does like the fact that there are multiple answers to the same problem. So I have been trying to understand if there is a common thread between them.

Yesterday, we watched an interesting TED talk about cancer and anti-angiogenic substances. As Dr. Li was talking, it dawned on me that many of the diets (all fruit, Vegan, Alkaline, Budwig, etc.) seem to have overlaps in the types of food that are 'allowed', and lo and behold, most of these are on the list of anti-angiogenic foods! The only diet that doesn't seem to fit in is the all meat diet that someone claims cured them. I am going to continue to think about this, but it is an interesting 'AH..HA'-moment for me.

Another point about advocating for yourself that should also be noted: First, let me say that anytime we have asked about anything, we never feel like we are asking a crazy question or that we are just 'stupid patients and Dr. Weber knows best'.

However, I do feel like if you DON'T ask about them, then they don't necessarily cross his mind. He will always take the time to explain the good and the bad about them and let you decide if that is something that you want to do.

For instance, there is a test that can be done in Greece (our understanding is that it is the only one in the world, but I may be wrong here) called the RGCC test - that will take a bunch of your blood, extract the cancer cells and make a hundred or more different cultures.

Then, they test it against a whole host of different substances such as garlic, curcumin, different types of chemo, etc. to see which ones work best for your specific cancer. It is costly, $2K, but it may be worth it to know.

One other thought on the topic of tests - it seems like the German medical system is much cheaper than the U.S. One of our good friends here had a full body scan and it only cost her €300. And, that was without any insurance. The same thing would have cost her over $3,000 in the US.

During our conversation, we got some more insight into Dr. Weber, the man himself. It seems that he used to live in the DDR before the Berlin wall came down. Back in the late 80's, he decided to try to get to West Germany. He had to make a very long trip through Poland, Czechoslovakia, Hungry, Austria, and finally to southern Germany. It sounded like a difficult trip. He didn't get to see his family (wife and 2 kids) for over a year until after the wall came down.

It was late in the day when he told us this, so we were feeling guilty keeping him from going home, but I have a 1,000 questions for him about that trip, what it was like living there, and why did he leave."

DAY ELEVEN AT MARINUS

JULY 19, 2018

"Alternative healing does not always offer a quick fix of a symptom, but it does offer a permanent healing that resonates beyond physical well-being. It creates a total uplift in attitude, enhanced spiritual awareness, and so much more that will change the way you appreciate life everyday. Embracing alternative healing by focusing on the cause and trusting the process as it unfolds will be a journey that can be trying or difficult at times, but it will always be extremely rewarding."
~ Alice McCal

West's post:
  "Day 11 -
  Ultrasound results are in!
  This morning we had another ultrasound with Dr. Helena. The good news is that the tumor is smaller now. It looks to be

about 2.6cm (just over 1 inch), which is a full centimeter smaller than when it was first measured (and .2 cm smaller than just last week!).

The better news is that the image is much 'lighter' which means, according to Dr. Helena, that the tumor is softer. I definitely could see the difference. Why is softer better? Here comes the geek again! Softer is better because it means there is more room for oxygen to get into the tumor. If you recall from one of my previous posts, cancer doesn't like oxygen. Therefore, if more oxygen can get into the tumor, then more suckers are going to leave. Good riddance! What we are doing is working and we are so thankful that we found this place.

This brings up another point. As we have spoken to more and more patients, we have realized this isn't a 'one and done' kind of treatment. We expect that we will have to come back again for follow up treatments, whether it be in 3 months, 6 months, or a year.

The good news - now that we know the ropes here, we have many more options. One that sounds kind of cool to me is to bring the kids with us. We can rent housing near the Klinik and some even have pools. I can definitely imagine taking the kids on hikes up the mountains, going to the Schwimmbad (local pool that looks more like a lake), riding bikes, playing with the cows, and riding horses, maybe even going skiing.

Today's Activities:

- NYC Ballet Workout (Self-directed)

- Breakfast (Oatmeal and Peppermint tea, both anti-angiogenic substances, and six red grapes, also an anti-angiogenic substance – we are easing into this)

- Reflexology

- Ozone Therapy IV drip (50 ml of blood removed, oxygenated by adding O3, then reintroduced to her body)

- Artemisinin IV drip (comes from a common garden plant artemesia or wormwood) – she seems to be getting an extra dose this week

- Vitamin C IV drip (and Vitamin B1, B6, and B12)

- Folic acid IV drip

- Thymus Peptide shot in the belly – immune system support

- Ultrasound

- Magnetic field therapy (Frema-magnetic field) focused on the tumor

- Bio mat pulsating magnetic fields and Oxygen

- Liver Pack

- Lunch (Salad and Sautéed Vegetables with brown rice)

- Hyperthermia - High heat treatment focused on the tumor

- *Voiceover Gig* in Rosenheim:

A sound engineer and personal friend from the VO biz contacted Leslie last week from the U.S. A long-standing client had moved up its fall promotion plans from August to this week. He wanted to let her know, to see if there was any way to record it from Germany. As it turns out, we have somehow figured out a way to make it happen!

We did some internet searches and were able to connect with a sound engineer who lives near Rosenheim was happens to be half German and half American!! He actually worked on the Big Apple Circus in NYC. His English was perfect, as was his German – we couldn't have asked for more! He hunted down a studio that could patch in the client, and he acted as a translator (thank the Lord for small miracles ☺).

So, we headed off to the studio in Rosenheim to record a couple of spots, with the client connected via a portal. Technology these days is amazing!

It went relatively well with only a few technical glitches, which the client wasn't even aware of! Leslie said it felt good to be working again – it made her feel 'normal' for a short time, and it was good to focus on something other than the cancer.

- Dinner

Since we were in Rosenheim, we decided to see if we could find a restaurant that will match our dietary needs. Lo and behold, we found an Indian restaurant (Ganesha Indisches

Restaurant) that had a decent Vegan menu. I was so excited -
one of my favorite foods is REAL Indian food!!

Maybe it was because we were tired of the same stir-fried
vegetables every night, but the food was outstanding. I couldn't
get enough, and our stomachs ached afterwards. Friday nights
are buffet nights at Marinus. There is little to nothing that we
can eat on the buffet, so we are probably going to trek to Rosenheim again and see if we can find some more yummy Vegan
food."

DAY TWELVE AT MARINUS

JULY 20, 2018

"Be willing to do whatever it takes to be a warrior for your own health." ~ **Jan Mundo**

West's post:
"Day 12 -
They moved where we sit in the dining room today, without letting us know!!!! Change is hard for me ☹!!

The new spot allows Leslie to see a 3-year-old girl who is here with her parents from Saudi Arabia. They make faces at each other throughout the meal. We both really miss Addison and Langdon, but at least she gets a little enjoyment from this little girl.

Leslie's energy level still isn't getting much better. We assume it is because her body is in overdrive healing the tumor. We are hoping to do some more exploring next week, energy and weather permitting.

Today's Activities:

- Yoga and Meditation (Self-directed)

- Breakfast (Grapes and an apple - both anti-angiogenic and no methionine)

- Massage

- Thymus Peptide shot in the belly – immune system support

- Mistletoe Extract Injection

- Magnetic field therapy (Frema-magnetic field) focused on the tumor

- Climbing a Mountain

Leslie seems to have some energy in the morning. We wanted to take advantage of it and took a walk up a mountain right behind the Klinik to a church that was built by Monks back in the 1800's. It certainly is not for the faint at heart, as it is a pretty steep incline.

On the way, we passed through a fairgrounds area (which seems out of place) where people come to rock climb. Then there is a steep set of stairs with caves dug into the granite with bars on them that look like jails. Some had religious icons in them, and others were empty. Beyond the church, there are a few look out spots that offer great views of the valley below.

- Liver Pack

- Lunch (Salad and Sautéed Vegetables with Quinoa)

- Hyperthermia - High heat treatment focused on the tumor

- Bio mat pulsating magnetic fields and Oxygen

- Shopping Trip to Rosenheim

Our trip to Rosenheim went so smoothly yesterday, we decided to see if we could make it a second day and do a little shopping in the area. Yay!!! (For those who don't know me, that was sarcastic about the shopping)

It was a beautiful day, but a little warmer than normal. Unfortunately, before we even left, Leslie had a headache, but she still wanted to go. This time, we jumped on our bikes and rode to the Brannenburg train station, which was really easy (downhill). The train was on time, but really packed - we were surprised to get seats.

We made it to Rosenheim with ease. As we started to walk towards the shopping area, Leslie got a little light-headed, so we stopped by an outdoor café and had a bottle of water. I guess gambling is more widely accepted in Germany as it was attached to a bookie! The cool water helped, and she felt better after a few minutes, so 'let the shopping begin'! Strangely, we found that all of the t-shirt sayings were written in English. We lasted for about 2 hours and were only able to buy a few things. Yay! (This one is not sarcastic)

- Dinner

Because of the meat and dairy-heavy buffet dinner at Marinus on Fridays, we made the decision to have dinner in Rosenheim again. I had researched a few places, but most of the places that offered Vegan menus were only open for lunch (do Vegan's eat dinner in Rosenheim??).

I found one other Indian restaurant that was near the train station. While we were at the café earlier in the day, we scoped it out (it was across the street). We decided to go back to the same place as last night because it was closer to the shopping area and we didn't want to have to figure out a new place. Besides, I don't like change!! Dinner was great again! The bike ride home wasn't as bad as we had expected - it was definitely better than the walk home the day before, though it was still uphill. Leslie was spent!

- Movie Night

Since we got home relatively early from Rosenheim, we went outside and watched *We're the Millers* as we were overlooking the mountains. It was okay until the WiFi started acting up again!"

YOUR BODY HAS THE POWER
TO HEAL

"The natural healing force within each of us is the greatest force in getting well." ~ **Hippocrates**

Leslie's post to the private FB group:

"I believe that if a cancer patient decides to do NOTHING - makes no changes to their lifestyle and chooses not to do a single treatment or therapy - regardless of the stage or form of the cancer, they are testing fate.

I also firmly believe that making radical changes to diet and lifestyle (clean living in both food and mind-body), along with non-toxic treatments like hyperthermia, IV-C drips, Ozone therapy, Mistletoe injections and the like, can HEAL the whole person without destroying the immune system.

I'm living proof that there are positive outcomes without chemo or radiation, and there are so many lovely people here at Marinus with similar stories of healing. It truly is an inspiring place to be.

Chris Wark gives some solid advice on reading scary cancer

studies (or headlines) and not believing everything as Ultimate Truth.

From Chrisbeatcancer.com: "The overall death rate for cancer has only improved about 5% in the last 60 years. And while most people don't know that shocking statistic exists (you're welcome), what they do know (including you, dear reader) is that cancer treatments have failed to save the lives of many people they love.

This is why, today, doctors are bombarded with questions from new patients about alternative therapies. I even asked my doctor about alternative options in 2004, to which he said,

" *"There are none. If you don't do chemotherapy, you're INSANE.""* ~ Chris Wark

DAY THIRTEEN AT MARINUS

JULY 21, 2018

*"At times our own light goes out and is rekindled by
a spark from another person.
Each one of us has cause to think deep gratitude of
those who have lighted the flame within us."*
~Author Unknown

West's post:

"Day 13 -

Today was the first day that I can say we were bored. Because we have been here so long, Leslie has slowly moved towards the morning timeslots for the scheduled treatments (i.e., Hyperthermia). She was done with all of her treatments before lunch and we had the whole afternoon to do whatever we wanted. Unfortunately, the rain had other ideas and kept us inside most of the day. Peeking our heads outside, we did get to see some of the low clouds covering the tops of the mountains, which was pretty cool.

We talked to the kids to hear about their adventures this

week and wish them a bon voyage as they head off to camp in Wisconsin tomorrow (Sunday). From what the kids reported, the good news is all of the activities, adventures, and experiences given to them through your generosity has kept them so busy they don't even notice we are gone.

The bad news is there is no way Leslie and I are going to be able to keep up the pace when we come back, and they are going to wish we would go away again. We can't say thank you enough for all of your support and help keeping our kids happy. You have gone way above and beyond!!"

**"Never stop believing because miracles happen
EVERY DAY." ~ Author Unknown**

West's post:

Day 14 –

"Today was another lazy day. Again, she was done before lunch and the weather was mostly still uncooperative. We are hoping Tuesday or Wednesday will be sunnier and maybe we can do some of the things we have wanted to do.

Leslie is starting to feel the difference in the tumor, meaning it feels softer and seems to be smaller. This certainly is helping our conviction.

We continue to hear great stories about people going home with great results. One of the women that Leslie befriended (because they could speak Dutch together ☺) is going home tomorrow. Her tumor has shrunk significantly, and Dr. Weber thinks that when she comes back in a few months it will be either gone or he will do the surgery to remove the small tumor. This friend was all smiles as we said goodbye!

We have been exchanging email addresses with lots of different people so that we can keep track of their progress. I hope that we will be able to keep in touch with these people and continue to hear their success stories.

We read books a portion of the day, and then watched a few movies from the collection downstairs. It was generally a lazy day.

Today's Activities:

- Yoga and Meditation (Self-directed)

- Breakfast (Vegetables and Fruits)

- Thymus Peptide shot in the belly – immune system support

- Magnetic field therapy (Frema-magnetic field) focused on the tumor

- Bio mat pulsating magnetic fields and Oxygen

- Hyperthermia - High heat treatment focused on the tumor. Leslie is getting even braver. She asked them to turn up the heat as she has heard others are at a higher setting. The nurse said they are only allowed to do that during the week when the Nurse Supervisor is here.

- Lunch (Spinach Soup and Vegetables with Potato Gnocchi – though much to our chagrin, we couldn't eat the Gnocchi)

- Afternoon Walk

We went out for a walk during one of the breaks in the clouds. It was a longer short walk and we tried to see 75 744, but no one was home.

- Dinner (More Spinach Soup, Potatoes and Vegetables)

- Movie Night

Last Vegas was pretty good - not a lot of belly laughs, but still entertaining.

Addicted to Love - we kept asking each other if we wanted to go to sleep (it was late, like 9:00 PM ;)), but we ended up watching the whole thing. It was ok, but not nearly as entertaining as *Last Vegas*."

DAY FIFTEEN AT MARINUS

JULY 23, 2018

*"If you just allow your body and mind to rest, the
healing will come by itself."*
~ **Thich Nhat Hanh**

West's post:
    "Day 15 -
    We had a bad sleeping night. Neither of us got a lot of sleep.
Leslie's restless leg syndrome kept her awake on and off all
night. The magnesium isn't helping. She has been having green
tea with ginger for dinner, so maybe it is the caffeine before bed.
We are hoping she gets more sleep tonight.
    Laundry Day! Yes, we get excitement out of little things
these days. Tomorrow, we will have clean clothes again.
    Leslie was done by midday again, so we had the afternoon
to ourselves. We spent most of the day outside either riding
bikes or reading under a tree looking at the mountains. It was a
very peaceful afternoon. There may have been a nap or two as
well.

We got one piece of disappointing news... It seems Dr. Weber went on vacation this week and we won't be able to speak to him before our departure on Sunday. There is another doctor here who we assume will talk to us before we leave about where we stand.

It really has been the only real disappointing aspect of the Klinik. From what I have heard from other patients, he does follow up with you after you leave, but it would have been nice to have a face-to-face discussion with him.

Today's Activities:

- Yoga and Meditation

- Breakfast (Avocado Salad, Oatmeal, Fruit)

The lady who serves/cooks for us, Kati, is very nice and funny! Since they technically don't have a Non-Gluten, Sugar Free, Vegan menu, we are always asking for something special, and they are very accommodating. As it turns out, Leslie and I always order the same thing as each other. Kati keeps teasing us about being two peas in a pod and unoriginal. Today, I crossed her up. Leslie had oatmeal, and I said 'No, thank you!' Kati's head nearly exploded! These are the things that entertain me these days.

- Massage

- Hyperthermia - High heat treatment focused on the tumor

- Blood draw for testing (5 vials for blood tests)

- Ozone Therapy IV drip (50 ml of blood removed, oxygenated by adding O_3, then reintroduced to her body)

- Artemisinin IV drip (comes from a common garden plant artemesia or wormwood)

- Folic acid IV drip (and Vitamin B1, B6, and B12)

- Selenium IV drip (essential trace mineral)

- Thymus Peptide shot in the belly – immune system support

- Magnetic field therapy (Frema-magnetic field) focused on the tumor

- Bio mat pulsating magnetic fields and Oxygen

- Liver Pack

- Lunch (Salad, Asparagus Soup and yup, you guessed it...Vegetables)

- Bike Trip to Town

Despite the weather, we decided to take a trip into town to get some snacks (nuts/berries) for the room. We are getting to know Brannenburg pretty well now, not that it is hard given its size. We went to a couple of different grocery stores and found some more nuts and a few blueberries to eat. We also stopped at a roadside strawberry stand that is shaped like a strawberry! We bought some freshly picked berries and wow, were they delicious!!

- Reading and Relaxing

The rain held off for the entire afternoon! We sat outside reading, and I may have fallen asleep at some point. I am one of those lucky people who can fall asleep without any effort. Leslie made fun of me because I guess I was trying to keep my book upright to give the illusion I was still reading.

- Dinner (More Asparagus Soup, this time with some potatoes and vegetables)

- Movie

Yes Man – I think we both had seen this before, but there were still a few good chuckles. Not sure I would say a full-on belly laugh.

The Switch – once again we watched to the end, but we really didn't enjoy it."

DAY SIXTEEN AT MARINUS

JULY 24, 2018

*"Laughter attracts joy and it releases negativity
and it leads to some miraculous cures."*
~ Steve Harvey

West's post:

"Day 16 -

Sleep was a little better last night, but Leslie woke early in the morning. We continue to look for solutions to this problem.

Yvette, the person who cleans our room, is so friendly and nice. She speaks exceptional English and uses many common slang phrases (with a German accent), which took me aback when we first spoke. Although she grew up in Germany, both of her parents are American. Anyway, she is the one who does our laundry.

She came to me today and asked when Leslie would be done. I enquired why, and she replied that she needed help determining whose clothes were whose. She was concerned they may have mixed up some clothes. I said that I should be able to help, and she was genuinely shocked. It is interesting that as advanced and liberal as they are in their thinking, they still have their stereotypes.

With the afternoon open, the sun shining, and the warm temperatures, we headed out to finally do some adventuring. We had a great time, but tired by the end of it.

Today's Activities:

- NYC Ballet

- Reflexology

- Breakfast (Oatmeal, Fruit)

- Hyperthermia - High heat treatment focused on the tumor

- Thymus Peptide shot in the belly – immune system support

- Magnetic field therapy (Frema-magnetic field) focused on the tumor

- Bio mat pulsating magnetic fields and Oxygen

- Liver Pack

- Lunch (Salad, Vegan Cream of Salsify, Potatoes and Vegetables)

- Wendelsteinbahn

We took a short bike ride to the bottom of the Wendelstein Cog Railway, which believe it or not, is a train that goes up to the top of the Wendelstein Mountain. It was a 25-minute train ride with lots of scenic views, a few scary 'don't look out the window' type moments, and a surprisingly large number of houses and cows very high up in the mountains. We passed a horse ranch that was giving kids riding lessons, which will make Addison so excited (I wish I had gotten a picture). At the top there is a restaurant (both cafeteria style as well as sit down), a church, and a trail that takes you up to the Observatory. I am happy to report that our patient was able to make the climb to the top! The good news was the whole way home was downhill, even the bike ride, which made her very happy.

- Dinner (Cream of Salsify Soup and Very Garlicky Vegetables)

We had some pretty good belly laughs at dinner tonight. It is hard to explain the situation, but let me just say we love a good dry wit, and Dr. Peter (a German MD who is having great success with his personal treatment here at Marinus) has wonderful timing with a few one-liners that sent us all into deep rolling laughs.

- Movie

This is 40 – We had seen this before, so we were expecting all of the jokes. We decided to try something else with not much success.

Friends with Money – We tried watching this, but it really wasn't all that interesting to us. We turned it off about halfway through.

Fun Mom Dinner – This looked like it was going to be funny, but alas, we struggled through it. In the end it wasn't funny."

DAY SEVENTEEN AT MARINUS

JULY 25, 2018

"The more consciousness you bring into the body, the stronger the immune system becomes. It is as if every cell awakens and rejoices. The body loves your attention. It is also a potent form of self-healing."
~ Eckhart Tolle (The Power of Now)

West's post:
  "Day 17 -
Sleep was better again last night, but that may have been more due to the Advil PM. She tries to avoid taking medications, but sleep is necessary for healing so she gave in, desperate for some quality shuteye. At this point, we will take whatever we can get.

  Despite our desire to wait as long as we could before the next ultrasound (we wanted to see as much improvement as possible), we had our last ultrasound today. We continue to get good news!

There were three pieces of good news today:

First, the tumor has shrunk again - it is now down to 2.4 cm. In addition, the doctor also said that some of that might be the hematoma from the biopsy, but she can't be sure.

It was interesting, as I think back on the doctor's reaction to the size - she seemed to be less excited about it than Leslie and I were. I think it is largely because all they have seen is the .4 cm reduction since we have been here. Leslie and I have seen a 1.2 cm reduction since the first measurements, and we are very excited about that!

Second piece of good news is it looks even softer than before, according to the doctor. As I was watching the ultrasound, I kept seeing a white spec in the middle of the tumor that faded in and out as she moved the probe slightly. I asked her about it, and she said it was a calcification. I am assuming it must be on the other side of the tumor because it wasn't consistent. We had never been able to see through the tumor before.

The third and probably best piece of news is that she believes the tumor is showing signs of necrosis (it has started to liquefy), meaning the cells inside the tumor are dying. I'll take that!!!

We then discussed what the next steps should be. Dr. Helena wanted us to consider taking the low dose Chemo pills, but we said as long as we continue to see improvements from these treatments and our diet, chemo wasn't interesting to us. She also suggested that we consider having the tumor removed. Again, we want to see how far we can get without surgery.

We settled on the following plan going forward:

She will continue to take Artemisinin and Mistletoe while we are at home. In 6-8 weeks, we'll have another ultrasound and send them the results. Depending on those results, they may suggest that we come back to Marinus in 2-3 months.

With the Vegan diet, the natural remedies, and pure deter-mination, we are going to 'Kick Cancer's Butt!'

Today's Activities included all of the typical treatments, and...

- Meeting with Head Nurse

After the ultrasound and meeting with the doctor, we had a follow up meeting with the Head Nurse to review the medicine going forward and ask any other questions. The one interesting takeaway is that all of these treatments should continue to work for the next 2-3 weeks after we leave.

- Reading and Relaxing

A thunderstorm rolled in during the afternoon, so we decided to go outside and sit under a tree and watch it, until we started getting wet. I love watching thunderstorms!"

DAY EIGHTEEN AT MARINUS

JULY 26, 2018

"I go to nature to be soothed, healed and have my senses put in order." ~ **John Burroughs**

West's post:
  "Day 18 -
  Sleep was allusive again for Leslie last night. The good news is that we only have 3 more nights here until she is back in her bed with her favorite pillow, where she can get comfortable.
  It was a very calm day here. Leslie's treatments were done by noon today, and we started to collect all of the medical supplies we are going to bring home - medications, syringes, etc. We took a quick jaunt down to the Schwimmbad for an afternoon dip, and laid around in the shade.

Today's Activities:

  • Reflexology

- Breakfast (Avocado Salad, Fruit)

- Hyperthermia - High heat treatment focused on the tumor

- Ozone Therapy IV drip (50 ml of blood removed, oxygenated by adding O3, then reintroduced to her body)

- Artemisinin IV drip (comes from a common garden plant artemesia or wormwood)

- Folic acid IV drip (and Vitamin B1, B6, and B12)

- Selenium IV drip (essential trace mineral)

- Thymus Peptide shot in the belly – immune system support

- Bio mat pulsating magnetic fields and Oxygen

- Magnetic field therapy (Frema-magnetic field) focused on the tumor

- Liver Pack

- Lunch (Salad, Herb Soup, Coconut Curry Vegetables and rice)

- Swimming at the Schwimmbad

Today was a warm day and perfect for swimming. We

pedaled down to the Schwimmbad, a lake-shaped swimming pool that is fed from a mountain stream and has an outlet to another waterway. The net result of this flow of water is that it is friggin' cold!! However, it is huge as pools go. Leslie only braved the cold up to her knees, but it was very refreshing (once you got in and used to it).

- Dinner (Roasted Vegetables)

- Movies:

Hangover – it was a fun watch that got a few belly laughs.
Crazy Ex-Girlfriend – we decided to try something new. We did not find it funny despite trying two different episodes."

INSPIRATION FOR HEALING

"The question is not whether we will die, but how we will live." ~ **Joan Borysenko**

While I was healing at Marinus, a friend made me aware of the HEAL summit, produced by Hay House.

It really was perfect timing - I was completely focused on healing myself using any holistic methods possible, and this summit offered many possibilities that I hadn't even known were out there.

There were so many inspirational speakers, but the interview with Joan Borysenko on July 26, 2018 really hit home.

I wish I could share it with you all, but the summit is long gone, and the links no longer work. However, I was able to find a description of the lesson and will include it below.

July 26: Joan Borysenko, Ph.D. – What Your Disease Is Trying to Teach You

"Lesson Description: In this heartfelt lesson, Joan Borysenko, Ph.D., teaches us to view disease as an initiatory rite of passage with hidden gifts. In fact, she explains it's our openness to *learning* from illness that foretells our fate... and, it is the power of love that we must lean upon as we traverse the path of illness and find within it *the joy of healing*.

You'll learn:

- A two-step plan for letting go of painful emotions
- How loneliness impacts your immune system
- The two emotions that keep you stuck and how to free yourself
- Why you need a higher cause to truly heal
- A 15-minute headache relief
- How self-love healed one woman of ALS"

Here is a short video excerpt from Joan's interview: A little test to see if your imagination can indeed effect your physiology, from the HEAL summit: *youtu.be/Ca4th_cxRpU*

In October, Hay House produced the ***Healing Cancer Summit***, with Kris Karr as the host. Of course, I was front and center for every interview, and learned so much!

If you ever get a chance to participate in a Hay House event, I highly suggest you do.

DAY NINETEEN AT MARINUS

JULY 27, 2018

"Life is amazing. And then it's awful. And then it's amazing again. And in between the amazing and the awful it's ordinary and mundane and routine. Breathe in the amazing, hold on through the awful, and relax and exhale during the ordinary. That's just living heartbreaking, soul-healing, amazing, awful, ordinary life. And it's breathtakingly beautiful." ~ **LR Knost**

West's post:

"Day 19 -

Second to last day of treatments!

Leslie described her sleep as 'spurty' (you will have to ask Leslie what that means!). I thought it was better because when I woke up a few times in the middle of the night, I didn't hear her rustling around.

This is the last business day of our stay here, meaning the

admin staff will be gone over the weekend. Therefore, we received our bill, and I was floored. Over the last 3 weeks at the Klinik, we received daily treatments and supplements, round the clock care (some patients needed it), a two-bed guest room onsite, 3 meals a day for 2 people plus snack time in the afternoon, 2 bike rentals, round-trip airport transfers for 2 people, laundry service, additional supplements to continue the treatment at home - and on top of it all, we have had some good results (priceless).

For all of that, the total cost was only $18K (also includes lodging and meals for the companion, an additional cost). If we had done outpatient care, it would have been $2-3K less expensive. We are so fortunate to have come across this place. We are very happy.

The one unfortunate thing we learned today was that our thoughts of coming here over the Christmas Holidays (assuming we haven't gotten rid of the tumor completely by then) with the kids won't work. They are closed from 12/17 through 1/7. Ah well, we will figure something out.

Today's Activities:

- Massage

- Breakfast (Avocado Salad, Fruit)

- Hyperthermia - High heat treatment focused on the tumor

- Thymus Peptide shot in the belly – immune system support

- Mistletoe Extract Injection

- Bio mat pulsating magnetic fields and Oxygen

- Magnetic field therapy (Frema-magnetic field) focused on the tumor

- Liver Pack

- Lunch (Salad, Vegetables and Quinoa)

- Yoga and Meditation – (self-directed)

- Dinner (Normally Buffet, but they made us a special Vegan meal)

- TV Shows

Will & Grace – we watched several episodes – as always it was pretty funny.

- Late Evening Walk

There was a full Lunar Eclipse last night in Brannenburg. We went out around 9:30 or so and searched for the moon. It took some time as there are so many trees, and it didn't pop up over the mountains until 9:45 or 10:00 pm. But it was pretty cool."

"We don't always choose what happens to us, but we can choose to see it as a positive, to believe it is for the best, and to use it to grow."
~ Khloe Kardashian

West's post:
   "Day 20 -
Our last full day at Klinik Marinus am Stein.
   It has been a great adventure! We have learned so much from the doctors, fellow patients, and our bodies. We are both going home healthier than when we got here, and even more determined that the path we are on is the correct one.
   These treatments are definitely showing signs of working, and we look forward to her next ultrasound in 6-8 weeks.
   I will let Leslie talk in detail about the emotional part of this journey, as I can't even come close to comprehending all of the emotions she has had to endure. However, watching her go from being scared and freaked out the day of the diagnosis to

now, where she is confident with ever-growing resolve that we can heal this with natural remedies has been awesome. She is an inspiration to me.

We leave early tomorrow morning and start the trek home. If everything goes as planned, we will be in Chicago by 2:30 pm and home shortly thereafter. We can't wait to see the kids and give them huge hugs!

Today's Activities:

- Yoga and Meditation – (self-directed

- Breakfast (Avocado Salad, Fruit)

- Hyperthermia - High heat treatment focused on the tumor

- Thymus Peptide shot in the belly – immune system support

- Bio mat pulsating magnetic fields and Oxygen

- Magnetic field therapy (Frema-magnetic field) focused on the tumor

- Lunch (Salad, Soup, and Vegetables)

- Walk

We took a walk after lunch to go say goodbye to 75 744.

Since it has been a while, he has found some friends, 75 150 and 75 151. Both are just as cute.

- Dinner (Sweet Potatoes and Vegetables)

- TV Shows

Will & Grace – again, it didn't disappoint.

We will continue to post here periodically as we get news. We can't say thank you enough to our family and friends who have made this so easy for us to be gone for 3 weeks.

From the little the kids have shared so far, they had an incredible time with all of the play dates, activities, and special outings.

We are forever in your debt. Thank you!"

GRATITUDE IS EVERYTHING

JULY 31, 2018

"Gratitude turns what we have into enough, and more. It turns denial into acceptance, chaos into order, confusion into clarity... it makes sense of our past, brings peace for today, and creates a vision for tomorrow." ~ **Melody Beattie**

Leslie's post to the private FB group:

"It is so good to be home!! What a joy to kiss my babies' sweet faces! And how fun that they made 'welcome home' signs and decorated the house! Thanks Auntie Jen for sending the banner kit to the kids!

I am so grateful for my healing journey at Marinus - it is an amazing place!

Furthermore, I am so grateful for many things here in Elmhurst as I continue my healing journey:

I am grateful for my phenomenal family and friends and their never-ending love and support. Shout out to Virginia for staying with the kids once they returned from camp on Saturday, until we got back home. And thanks again to Sarah for getting them home safely after a fun-filled week at camp (with a stop at a lake, I hear!)

I am grateful for Vegan Indian food in La Grange on Sunday night, so we didn't have to cook - there may actually be possibilities for us to eat out on occasion!

Grateful for my bathtub! Oh, what a joy to slip into a hot bath on Sunday night, filled with Epsom salts and lavender oil... I promptly fell asleep (yes, IN the tub...), and knew I was ready for bed even though it was only 8 pm in Chicago and we'd barely gotten the kids off to their rooms.

I am grateful for my comfy bed and supportive pillow!! AHHHH... and my extra long bed where I can stretch out and really get comfortable.

I am grateful for temperature control! It makes it so much easier to sleep when the room is cool and comfortable. And blackout shades!!! I loved waking up to the birds singing in Germany, but 5 am comes early when the windows are open and there are no curtains...

I am grateful for soft carpeting to do my meditation and 'legs up the wall' before bed - I was getting some serious rug burns on my elbows in Germany.

I am grateful to have a fully stocked kitchen at our disposal! And so grateful to have a husband who is rocking this Vegan cooking! West is going to be the next celebrity Vegan chef - mark my words!

Grateful for our new masticating juicer! West made me fresh wheat grass juice yesterday, and it was delicious and incredibly healing. Now I don't have to make numerous trips to Whole Foods every day.

And grateful that my husband is home to help me on this journey. It turns out things really do happen for a reason.

Grateful for cuddles from my kids! I hit a wall last night around 6 pm (jetlag doesn't suit me well. I remember it always took me a ridiculously long time to acclimate when traveling to and from Holland in the '90s... it's all coming back to me now...), so we curled up on the couch together and watched *Ellen's Game of Games* and laughed. As Addison said, 'remember mom - laughter is the best medicine!'

Grateful for a clear schedule, so when I can't sleep for several hours in the middle of the night, I can rest assured that I don't have to get up in the morning to rush off to anything, and can peacefully fall back asleep without worry...

Life is GOOD."

MAKING SELF-CARE A PRIORITY

"With every act of self-care your authentic self gets stronger, and the critical, fearful mind gets weaker. Every act of self-care is a powerful declaration: I am on my side, I am on my side, each day I am more and more on my own side."
~ Susan Weiss Berry

Returning home from 3 weeks in Germany proved to be challenging. After all, my only true responsibility at Marinus was to focus on healing. But at home, it was back to real life and all of the obligations that came along with it.

Acclimating back into family life was tricky... especially with the kids on summer break. I love my kids so much, but let's be honest - parenting can be stressful!! The sibling fights, the early tweenager meltdowns, the slamming doors, the boy humor. Especially when you add in jetlag...our fuses were shorter than normal. My nerves were feeling worn.

What truly was lacking was a quiet house. I was finding it very difficult to carve out space to find peace and time to myself to do the things I needed to do to continue healing.

It's such a balancing act, certainly for a parent trying to heal from a devastating disease. But I fully recognize that it can be challenging for any of us to put self-care at the top of our daily to-do list.

Cancer is a powerful motivator. It was now a matter of life or death, and I found it much easier to say no to so many requests of my time. I knew that I needed to do everything in my power to make sure I was still around for my kids next year and for many years beyond that - which meant, for now, it would be less Monopoly and Barbies, and more sauna time, yoga and meditation.

And I had to do it without "Mommy guilt" - because, honestly, guilt is completely pointless and diminishes any positive effects of your efforts. LET IT GO.

Wouldn't it be great if each of us could put ourselves FIRST without needing the scary wake up call?

Perhaps my journey can be a lesson for others - inspiration for you to make some changes in your life, starting today.

Schedule a massage (so good for blood circulation and stress reduction), take a detox bath, spend 15 minutes meditating every evening, get to bed 30 minutes earlier, take a walk after dinner with your kids and really connect, or call that friend who always makes you smile.

The list goes on and on. Pick something that really makes you feel GOOD. And then do it again... and again. And soon, being good to yourself will become a habit.

You deserve to be healthy and happy. And you make that choice each and every day.

CHOOSE PEACE. CHOOSE HAPPINESS. CHOOSE YOU.

"Showing gratitude is one of the simplest yet most powerful things humans can do for each other."
~ Randy Pausch

Leslie's post to the private FB group:
  "GRATITUDE!

- I'm thankful for the guy at Whole Foods who was willing to sell me an entire tray of living wheat grass! Daily shots of health – hallelujah!
- Thankful to my husband who is now making the most amazing Vegan foods! He made almond butter and almond milk from SCRATCH, and it's delicious!!
- Thankful for the homegrown tomatoes from the Emerson garden, which Chef West made into a phenomenal marinara sauce and served it over crispy polenta cakes.

- Thankful for Wellness House, so I have a peaceful and supportive haven to which I can escape when needed. ❤
- Thankful for my amazing mom, Pat - the kids had a great time with you, as always!
- Thankful for my sweet friend, Caryn, for taking the kids to lunch and swimming - they had a blast with you and Gina!
- Thankful for my Diva sister, Barri, and her never-ending rescues and fun outings for the kids!!
- Thankful for walking buddies, Vanitha & Angie, (and the sugar/gluten free Vegan meal from Daily Harvest!) and 'gabbing over lunch' buddies, Barri & Jen.
- Thankful for the GORGEOUS bouquet of flowers from Farmgirl that arrived on my doorstep from Elliott and Rebecca!

ARTEMISININ & MISTLETOE

"Nature itself is the best physician."
~ Hippocrates

I realized that healing naturally would never be possible if I wasn't 100% committed, and I was fortunate that my husband and kids understood that concept and supported me. Healing the cancer would be my number ONE priority.

Now that I was back home and starting to figure out how to find some peace in the midst of the often crazy family life, I needed to commit to a consistent schedule for each of the holistic approaches that would continue to heal me.

I began taking the Artemisinin pills daily that Dr. Weber had sent home with me from Germany, as well as twice-weekly Mistletoe injections subcutaneously in my abdomen.

ARTEMISININ

The *Artemisia annua* plant contains chemical compounds considered to have anticancer activity. Artemisinin is a natural derivative of *Artemisia annua*, and artesunate is a prescription medication derived from *Artemisia annua*.

"The National Cancer Institute conducted a study with 55 different cancer cell lines to evaluate their response to in vitro treatment with artesunate. In this study, several cancer cells demonstrated susceptibility to the compound, including breast, prostate, ovary, colon, kidney, central nervous system, and melanoma cells...They concluded that (it) inhibited the proliferation of the cancer cells, arrested them in the G0/G1 phase, and with an increased concentration of the drug, they managed to induce apoptosis."

This paper explains the current thinking behind treating cancer with Artemisinin:

www.researchgate.net/profile/Narendra_Singh16/publication/8382373_Artemisinin_induces_apoptosis_in_human_cancer_cells/links/54c14b750cf2dd3cb9584019.pdf

MISTLETOE EXTRACT

The liquid extract of the mistletoe plant has been used in Europe for close to a century to improve quality of life and improve survival in patients with cancer. Mistletoe injections are currently among the most widely used complementary cancer treatments in Europe.

John Hopkins: Are mistletoe injections the next big thing in cancer therapy?

www.hub.jhu.edu/magazine/2014/spring/mistletoe-therapy-cancer

"An increasing number of studies have reported anticancer activity of mistletoe extracts on breast cancer cells and animal models. Various studies on mistletoe therapy for breast cancer patients revealed similar findings concerning possible benefits on survival time, health-related quality of life, remission rate, and alleviating adverse reactions to conventional therapy."

www.hindawi.com/journals/bmri/2014/785479

"*Mistletoe injections have demonstrated effective results in several trials based in Europe, extending life and reducing symptoms associated with cancer.

*Most people will either have a personal experience or know someone who has cancer as an estimated 1.7 million new cases of cancer will be diagnosed in the U.S. in 2018; the most common of which are breast, lung, prostate and colorectal cancers.

*Suzanne Somers, actress, author and health advocate, was diagnosed with breast cancer in 2011 and chose to use natural strategies, including mistletoe extract, to successfully treat her disease.

*Although chemotherapy may make breast cancer aggressive and more likely to spread, other natural treatment options may offer similar, if not better, results."

www.articles.mercola.com/sites/articles/archive/2018/11/07/mistletoe-extract-tumor-treatment.aspx

DAILY GREEN JUICE

"Remember that every single green drink you create is an investment in your quality of life – now and always." ~ Kris Carr

While at Marinus for those 3 weeks, I really began missing my daily fresh-pressed green juice and wheatgrass shots that we would get at the Whole Foods juice bar, near our home. I could hardly believe it myself...boy, I had to choke down that very first wheatgrass shot!

However, it does grow on you over time, and I knew how chock full of nutrients each sip of this green miracle liquid was. It was now a priority to get as many of these powerhouse phytochemicals into my body as often as possible to strengthen my immune system.

So I begged West to order a juicer that would be waiting for us once we got back home, so we could fresh press our delicious healing green juices at home every morning!

He did the research on different types and different brands

of juicers, and ultimately chose the Omega Masticating Juicer. What is a masticating juicer, you may ask? Well, it slowly presses the juice from almost anything using an auger to slowly crush the produce of choice. This means that your juice will retain more of the beautiful nutrients, and you get *more* juice from the produce, too! Another perk: it can also make home-made almond butter!

A centrifugal juicer, in contrast, uses blades to shred the produce. It also generates more heat than a slow juicer, which can damage valuable components of the juice. You get a lot more waste in the end, but it is a faster method to get to the finished product. These are the types of juicers you'll typically find in a commercial juice bar.

Since our main focus is healing, we figured the more nutrients, the better! Quality over speed!

Yes, it takes dedication to do this every morning - to clean the fruits and vegetables, to chop them, to clean the juicer afterwards. But it's well worth it to get that flood of vibrant vitamins and minerals, a veritable cornucopia of health in a glass!

It's best to drink your green juice on an empty stomach to make the most of this amazing drink. Since the fiber has been removed, your body gets a break from digestion and the true goodness of the produce rushes to your cells, giving you a tremendous boost first thing in the morning. What a way to start the day! ☺

To get the most nutrition out of your juice, it's best to drink it immediately after it's been cold pressed. The enzymes in those gorgeous fruits and veggies begin to break down as soon as they hit the air.

We typically make our green juice out of the following: wheatgrass, kale, romaine, spinach, celery, cucumbers, carrots, green apple and lemon. But we'll often add in other things that we've got in the kitchen – changing it up keeps things interesting! Sometimes midday we'll throw together a carrot/apple/ginger juice, or as a special treat, a 'green lemonade' (just green apples and lemon).

We've started giving Langdon, our 8-year old son, a big glass of green juice every morning, and now he actually asks for it! (ok... maybe we add in a little watermelon or orange to make it more appealing to a kid ;)). He gets the equivalent of 10-15 servings of fruits and veggies in that one glass – no gummy bear vitamins necessary for this guy!

I've also taken to doing a 48-hour juice fast once a month to clear out any bad habits (it revives your taste buds and reduces cravings), and to give the body a break from digestion.

Did you know that 70% of your energy is used on the 3 stages of digestion? Imagine the healing that can happen when that energy can be focused elsewhere.

When we support our bodies and the work that it is meant to do, health is a wonderful side effect. Create space to allow your body's innate wisdom to do its work.

YOU are your own best healer!

JUST MOVE

"When you really want something, you will find a way. When you don't really want something, you'll find an excuse." ~ **Rachel Hollis**

As we all know, daily exercise is essential for a healthy body and a peaceful mind, but it is especially important for those of us healing from a chronic disease. We should all aim to get at least 30 minutes of physical activity every single day – no excuses!

Get outside and take a brisk walk after dinner or during your lunch break (this will also make you more productive in the afternoon without needing the candy bar or coffee pick me up!), park at the farthest spot to get more steps in, take the stairs instead of the elevator (and then go back down and do it again!), do 15 minutes of sit ups and push ups before you hop in the shower in the morning, or get your butt to a class that will motivate you.

My exercise class of choice is yoga. I'm a member at Yoga By

Degrees, which allows me to take any class I want, at any time, at any of their 6 locations. I try to get there at least 3 or 4 times a week, and I miss it when I'm not able to fit it in.

It's a wonderful place focused on the *total* experience of yoga, so it's not only about moving my body – it also helps calm my spirit and quiet my mind (a big bonus!). Many classes are also heated to varying degrees (thus the 'by degrees' part of their name), which allows for a deeper cleanse of the body as well as many other benefits.

> *"Besides getting our minds to slow down and improving our overall mental health, yoga has numerous physical benefits as well. A regular hatha yoga practice helps increase your body's flexibility, helps improve posture, helps relieve and heal back aches, helps reduce blood pressure, helps lower cholesterol and decrease body fat, helps prevent injury and helps to stabilize blood glucose levels... In addition, a regular yoga practice will strengthen, lengthen and tone the muscles in the body. Yoga also promotes better sleep and improves digestion and, often times, metabolism."* ~ Yoga By Degrees

If I can't make it to a class because of a busy work schedule or family obligations, I do my best to fit in a 30-minute yoga or ballet session at home. Pick some of your favorite postures that make your body feel good and go for it!

If you're newer to yoga, there are also wonderful videos online that offer guidance for free. While I was in Germany, I often turned to "Yoga By Adriene" for some inspiration – I love her energy, and she's good at breaking things down.

I've got some awesome health-minded friends who are always willing to try something new with me, and one of those friends is Stephanie. I convinced her to join me at Morton Arboretum for a unique yoga experience hanging from the trees! AERIAL YOGA in a tree – how fantastic is that!?!

STRESS BECOMES A FACTOR

AUGUST 15, 2018

"Emotional pain cannot kill you, but running from it can. Allow. Embrace. Let yourself feel. Let yourself heal." **~ Vironika Tugaleva**

I had an immensely stressful life event occur on August 15 that completely changed the course of my healing. I won't go into the details, but it shook me to my core, and I felt the ripple effect of the stress it created in my body for months to come... it became even more difficult to focus on healing my body, and this would be reflected in my test results.

"Evidence from experimental studies does suggest that psychological stress can affect a tumor's ability to grow and spread... Studies in mice and in human cancer cells grown in the laboratory have found that the stress hormone norepinephrine, part of the body's fight-or-flight response system, may promote angiogenesis and metastasis."

www.cancer.gov/about-cancer/coping/feelings/stress-fact-sheet

"Stress fuels cancer spread by triggering master gene."
www.medicalnewstoday.com/articles/265254.php

SQUARE ONE

AUGUST 16, 2018

"If my diet and lifestyle choices, and my attitude
and my emotions have contributed to me being
sick, then what if I change everything?
What could happen? Maybe my body can heal."
~ Chris Wark

I begin Chris Wark's Square One Program.

A little about Chris: Chris Wark was diagnosed with stage IIIc colon cancer in 2003. After surgery, he opted-out of chemo and used nutrition and natural therapies to heal. Today, 16 years later, he is healthy, strong, and still cancer-free!

He shares his story in full detail and does a lot of survivor interviews, which are not only inspirational, but also empowering. There is so much valuable information in his program - not just for healing cancer, but also preventing it and many other chronic Western diseases.

I purchased this program for myself, and shared it with a good friend who was healing from cancer. It has been very helpful, keeping me focused on what is truly important on this journey.

I dedicated time for each module and incorporated many of his suggestions into my healing protocol. I also joined the Facebook support group and am still moderately active in this group today.

IV THERAPY

"Science, especially natural and medical science, is always undergoing evolution, and one can never hope to have said the last word upon any branch of it." ~ **Alphonse Laveran**

My Integrative Medicine doctor recommended that I visit a place about 40 minutes away that offers high-dose vitamin C IV infusions with selenium, B complex and Glutathione, similar to what I was getting at Marinus in Germany. It ain't cheap ($220 per infusion), but at least I feel like I'm not slowing down too much on the treatment side because of it. I can't let this tumor think it has the upper hand!!

August 18, 2018 – I start IV treatments – first visit was 25 grams of vitamin C. They also drew blood to run a test to make sure my body could handle higher amounts of C. If so, we can raise it at future infusions.

"The study shows that vitamin C breaks down easily, generating hydrogen peroxide, a so-called reactive oxygen species that can damage tissue and DNA. The study also shows that tumor cells are much less capable of removing the damaging hydrogen peroxide than normal cells."

www.sciencedaily.com/releases/2017/01/170109134014.htm

More good news about the power of IV vitamin C:

www.natureworksbest.com/vitamin-c-cancer-therapy/

High doses of IV vitamin C have been shown to improve *outcomes of chemotherapy and radiation as well:*

www.medicalnewstoday.com/articles/316643.php

INFARED SAUNAS

AUGUST 21, 2018

"The best and most efficient pharmacy is within your own system." ~ **Robert C. Peale**

Hallelujah! West installed a far infrared sauna in our basement (2nd best option to hyperthermia), and I'm now making daily visits. Farewell, damaged cells!! Hello, healthy new cells!!

"Infrared sauna treatments are exceptionally promising because of the selective toxicity they have on cells. In a nutshell, the hyperthermic effects of infrared radiation are only harmful to malignant cells... Dr. Sahni told us that normal healthy cells are essentially immune to infrared radiation, while cancer cells are hyper-thermically challenged: ...by exposing your body to that heat, you're selectively killing or eradicating those less viable cells, those cancer cells, without hurting your normal cells. And so a far infrared sauna is useful because it can help you sweat, excrete toxins, and in theory, eliminate cancer cells which can't survive the heat."

Another study published in the *Journal of Cancer Science*

and Therapy found that after just 30 days of infrared treatment, tumor-infected mice saw reductions in their cancerous masses of up to *86%* – even with low-temperature infrared exposures of as little as 77 degrees Fahrenheit (25 Celsius).

And if that isn't enough, another study out of Japan found that infrared-induced, whole-body hyperthermia helped strongly inhibit the growth and spread of breast cancer cells in mice, without causing any harmful side effects." https://thetruthaboutcancer.com/infrared-sauna-benefits/

I have GOT to make time for the various healing treatments in my daily life! It's challenging with day-to-day responsibilities, but it's so very important and I can't let myself get distracted...

*When I shared this in the private Facebook support group, some wise friends had some inspiring words for me:

N: "Let me just share this from an old guilty working mom mindset - if you had a business meeting or a VO gig - you could not be any place else but there - right? The answer is yes! And I witnessed it first hand because we just recorded together for three hours - Couldn't take a call or text etc. - the trick is to use the same mindset to frame your 'healing sessions', whatever they may be. It's as, no, more important. When you are recording, you have made arrangements to cover the kids and are not worried about losing the next gig - same applies - it's mindset girlfriend - here to help any way I can to free up the time you need."

Me: "Excellent point - I need to 'book' myself for these treatments, and not let anything get in the way."

N: "Yes exactly! Start small and it will become a wonderful habit."

L: "Great way to look at it. At work, we are encouraged to block time on our calendars for personal development. This is even more important."

J: "MUST. MAKE. TIME. TO. HEAL. I'm going to set an alarm each day to check in on you on this - pick your time."

It eventually became a daily habit: jumping on the rebounder, dry skin brushing to move the lymphatic system (more on these other approaches in future posts), infrared sauna, meditation, and a liver pack or detox bath at night. My health and healing has become THE priority.

MOVE THAT LYMPH!

"When a plant's leaves are turning brown you don't paint the leaves green. You look at the cause of the problem. If only we treated our bodies the same way." ~ **Dr. Frank Lipman**

I was now a big fan of Kris Carr, and was truly amazed and inspired by the radical changes she made in her life after getting her cancer diagnosis. She has successfully managed her stage 4 cancer, and has been a champion cancer THRIVER for over 16 years!!

I purchased her *Crazy Sexy Cancer* DVD and have watched it (including all bonus features) many times. One of her recommendations was to jump on a rebounder daily to get the lymphatic system moving. This assists your body in clearing out any toxins, including any cancer cells that have died off - Good riddance!!

It's so important for us to let our body do all of the amazing, miraculous things that it was built to do, and make sure we aren't getting in its way. And sometimes, just sometimes, we need to give it a little nudge in the right direction... with some movement!

"The lymphatic system is the metabolic garbage can of the body. It rids you of toxins such as dead and cancerous cells, nitrogenous wastes, fat, infectious viruses, heavy metals, and other assorted junk cast off by the cells. The movement performed in rebounding provides the stimulus for a free-flowing system that drains away these potential poisons.

Unlike the arterial system, the lymphatic system does not have its own pump. It has no heart muscle to move the fluid around through its lymph vessels. There are just three ways to activate the flow of lymph away from the tissues it serves and back into the main pulmonary circulation. Lymphatic flow requires muscular contraction from exercise and movement, gravitational pressure, and internal massage to the valves of lymph ducts. Rebounding supplies all three methods of removing waste products from the cells and from the body."

www.vitalitymagazine.com/article/rebounding-good-for-lymphatic-system

"The health effects of rebounding happen at a cellular level and at a higher rate than other forms of exercise. Rebounding can make the difference in your health and happiness by increasing your blood flow, loosening your tight muscles, flushing your lymphatic system, releasing endorphins, and clearing your mind. The rebounding action is impact free, it removes the impact of tension and stress on your body, and it's really enjoyable!"

www.beatcancer.org/blog-posts/how-rebounding-exercise-affects-your-immune-system

I purchased a sturdy, yet inexpensive rebounder on eBay, and it does the job! And the kids enjoy the rebounder, too! Sometimes I have to fight to get my time on it. Any excuse to get us all moving!

BRUSH THAT SKIN

"The cure of many diseases is unknown to physicians... because they are ignorant of the whole. For the part can never be well unless the whole is well." ~ **Plato**

Dry Skin Brushing... what the heck is it?? And what's the point?

Dry skin brushing is an ancient Ayurvedic technique, aiding the body's lymphatic system in removing the metabolic waste and environmental toxins floating around our bodies. And when you're healing from cancer, clearing out the toxins is a number one priority! Healing my body had become such a focus in my life, and I was willing to add in any natural methods that came across my path.

The lymphatic system is this incredible pathway throughout our bodies. Though often overlooked, it's an important part of our body's immune system, and can facilitate healing when done correctly. If this pathway gets clogged with toxic sludge, the body can't work efficiently. Just like if your sink or toilet gets clogged – you must clear it in order for waste to move out.

Lymph nodes are the filtration stops in this intricate web. Lymph nodes are located in various places in our bodies like the armpits, the neck, and the groin, and these amazing little nodes help to carry the toxins and sludge away, so problems don't develop. This is why the doctors look for swollen lymph nodes that will show if we're "fighting" something like a cold. The toxins are then sent to the heart and on to other elimination organs like the liver, so they can leave the body.

For some reason, the lymph system doesn't have a pump like the cardiovascular system does (the heart), so it is essential that we do what we can to help move things along.

Exercise can help stimulate lymphatic drainage, which is why it's important to get in a walk every day or jump on that rebounder.

Another important way to help stimulate your lymphatic system is brushing your skin, the largest organ we have. The lymphatic system is just below the surface of the skin; so gently brushing it with a natural-bristle brush will move things along. But brushing in the right direction is a key element, so the lymph fluids sail to the nodes and are able to be eliminated properly. Basically, brushing towards the heart is a good rule.

I always do my dry skin brushing routine immediately before getting into the infrared sauna, but you can also hop in the shower afterwards to wash off everything that was brought to the surface. In fact, I hop in the shower after the sauna anyway! Gotta wash away all the yuckies that come out!

Better lymphatic circulation may lead to other health perks as well, including improved digestive and respiratory function, smoother skin, less cellulite and more energy. So why not start today? ☺

TALK THERAPY

"The greatest weapon against stress is our ability
to choose one thought over another."
~ William James

I was dealing with a lot in my life, and it only got worse after that momentous event that happened in August – all of the stress was wearing on me, and I needed an outlet.

I found a wonderfully caring therapist who I began seeing weekly. I had found a safe space to talk about everything that was weighing on my mind. It was only an hour, but it was a lifesaver.

Sometimes we need someone outside of our inner circle who can just listen, and perhaps when appropriate, offer a new perspective. And sometimes we don't even need input – we often figure out exactly what we need just by saying it out loud.

From Psychology Today:

"Why do experts advise *talking* after a crisis regardless if it's small, big, personal, or national? Because it's one of our natural, built-in, therapeutic capacities. We use our words to express what we want and need and the same should be for our feelings....

Talking can help us in many ways, especially if our trauma or problem is on-going, unexpected, or doesn't have an easy answer.

Reasons to Talk

1. It gives us a sense of 'doing' something. By talking, we are doing something active not passive, and we are reaching out for a connection.
2. Talking gives us an opportunity to 'hear' ourselves and 'listen' to ourselves. It gives us an opportunity to adjust our thoughts and feelings. Hearing ourselves say, 'I can't take another day of this' might lead us to add, 'Unless I get help', or 'But I will'.
3. Lastly, talking teaches us that thoughts and feelings are usually less ominous when we say them out loud to others versus thinking about them privately.

If you need to talk, reach out and find someone who will listen. However, *not any listener* will do. This is especially true if your stress is ongoing, unexpected, and doesn't have an easy answer, like an emotional loss from a miscarriage, a job-related problem, a friendship crisis, or a health problem."

I AM HEALTHY. I AM HEALING. I AM HEALED

"I have come to believe that caring for myself is not self indulgent. Caring for myself is an act of survival." ~ **Audre Lorde**

I was also making use of the amazing offerings for cancer patients at Wellness House in Hinsdale. Their mission is simple – to better the lives of people living with cancer and the people close to them. And their services are offered at absolutely no cost to anyone touched by cancer.

What a blessing to have found this healing place!

Besides the support groups, yoga and meditation classes, and family events that I participated in, I began doing Reiki sessions at Wellness House, and it was so very helpful to my state of mind.

If you're not familiar with Reiki, allow me to give you a brief overview: Reiki is an ancient holistic therapy aimed at restoring the natural energetic balance in the patient's body. It is believed to aid in healing, reduce stress, release emotional blockages, and induce relaxation.

The patient, fully clothed, gets into a comfortable position, usually lying on a table. A trained practitioner places their hands on or over specific areas of the patient's body, and transfers the universal energy known as 'chi' or 'prana' from their hands into the patient.

I'll be honest – when my primary doctor at Elmhurst Memorial Hospital suggested that I try this therapy, I was skeptical. Would it truly be helpful? But in my first session, I experienced something quite intriguing to me.

My eyes were closed, and at her urging, I repeated the following mantra to myself as she worked – "I am healthy, I am healing, I am healed".

She slowly moved around the table, concentrating her energy at different places around my body. At times, I could feel heat coming from her hands, and at other times I felt a vibration over the area.

She then came around to the right side of my body, where the tumor was located. I suddenly felt the strangest sensation, as if she were gently pressing against the tumor site with her hands. It didn't hurt, but it did give me pause.

Emotions started stirring, and I began to tear up. The Reiki master, a kind and compassionate woman, encouraged me to allow myself to feel these emotions, and not to push them down or try to control them.

I tried hard not to let my extreme vulnerability get in the way of this experience, which was a challenge. Once I was able to let go, I began sobbing uncontrollably. It was raw and slightly scary, but incredibly cleansing. Clearly, I had been trying to hold things together, and I was bursting at the seams.

Once the session was done, I asked her if she was indeed

touching me at any point during the therapy. She said no... her hands were always several inches above or outside of my body. I told her about the pressure I had felt on and around the tumor, and how certain I was that I felt her hands on me. She explained that it was the energetic force being driven into the area of my body where it was most needed. Wow... I was now a believer.

66 *"According to practitioners, energy can stagnate in the body where there has been physical injury or possibly emotional pain. In time, these energy blocks can cause illness.*

Energy medicine aims to help the flow of energy and remove blocks in a similar way to acupuncture or acupressure. Improving the flow of energy around the body, say practitioners, can enable relaxation, reduce pain, speed healing, and reduce other symptoms of illness." ~ *Medical News Today*

MORE HEALING THERAPIES

"Create space to allow your body's innate wisdom
to do its work. You are your own best healer."
~ Sarah Raymond

I was also able to add a few more calming self-care elements to my life.

My Integrative Medicine doctor suggested that I schedule a session of Guided Imagery with Pastor Don through the hospital. Don is such a kind-hearted man, soft spoken and loving – everything you'd want when you're trying to find peace.☺

I sat in a comfortable chair with my eyes closed, and listened to his calming voice. He guided me to my "happy place", aiding me in painting pictures in my mind that would be relaxing, and ended by leading me in some positive affirmations. It was a pleasant experience, and I would encourage others to give it a try.

He encouraged me to record our session on my phone, so I

could replay it whenever I needed to return to this peaceful place in my mind. I used it often...

I also discovered that NEXT yoga in Elmhurst offered sessions on a biomat! This was one of the treatments that I received in Germany, so I was thrilled to find something available so close to home. I would lie on the warm mat in a dimly lit yoga studio while listening to my recorded guided imagery, and it was very relaxing.

It turns out it wasn't exactly the same kind of biomat as the high-tech version at the German clinic, but it was still beneficial, especially to calm my frazzled nerves. What they used at NEXT was an amethyst biomat, rather than a Bemer biomat (more on this later).

"The Biomat is an FDA licensed medical device that combines state of the art Far Infrared light and Negative Ion technology with the healing power of Amethyst crystal. ... Many have experienced numerous benefits from far infrared and negative ion technology, including: Improved circulation and cardiovascular function."

www.biomathealth.com/what-is-the-biomat

AMAZING GREEN GRASSES

"Everything in your life is a reflection of a choice you have made. If you want a different result, make a different choice." ~ **Author Unknown**

Now that we were doing all of our own juicing at home, it seemed prudent to purchase large quantities of wheatgrass instead of the tiny little boxes that get you through one or two juices at a time.

I couldn't continue to beg Ed at the store to sell me trays of the amazing green grasses, so I asked him who their supplier was. He told me it was Chicago Indoor Garden – so I did a little search, found their info, and reached out to them, asking if it might be possible to purchase trays of wheatgrass directly from them. Perhaps I could meet their truck at Whole Foods when they're doing the typical delivery.

My contact was so kind, and happens to live in the 'burbs not far from me, so she offered to drop my order off on my doorstep on her way home! There was an additional fee for delivery, but I was excited to get still-living wheatgrass delivered to my door every week! ☺

Since they were making the trip, I asked what other products they offered? They only grow wheatgrass and sprouts (no lettuces or veggies – darn). We'd been learning about the incredible nutritional profile of certain sprouts such as broccoli sprouts, pea sprouts and sunflower sprouts, and lo and behold, they grow all of those as well!

Chicago Indoor Garden began delivering trays of wheatgrass once a week at the end of August, and we immediately started adding them to our daily juice.

UNEXPECTED DERAILMENT

"As my sufferings mounted I soon realized that there were two ways in which I could respond to my situation — either to react with bitterness or seek to transform the suffering into a creative force. I decided to follow the latter course."
~ Martin Luther King Jr

If you recall, I had been to a nearby clinic for my first high-dose vitamin C IV infusion in August. They could only do 25 grams until the blood test results came back and hopefully showed that I did not have the genetic mutation (G6PD) that could make this treatment dangerous.

Sadly, they called me before that 2nd session to tell me that there was a problem with the blood that had been drawn, and they couldn't complete the test. Apparently, my blood had been mishandled, as I would later learn, and could no longer be used for the G6PD test. I was told they'd have to limit the infusion to

25 grams again, and take another sample of blood to rerun the test.

Ok, no big deal, I guess. What's one more week? It was more frustrating than anything. I was anxious to increase the dosage since anything less than 50 grams isn't thought to be effective for treating cancer, though it would still boost my immunity.

However, in the middle of that 2nd session, the doctor at the infusion clinic approached me in my chair, while I had a needle in my arm and an IV bag dripping above my head. He sauntered over with his collar up, papers in his hand, and began speaking with a cocky attitude, "Your liver enzymes are elevated. The cancer has spread to your liver." Yeah, his bedside manner could use a little improvement.

This news took me by surprise. "I thought you weren't able to run the tests??" He said that he thinks the blood was left out while waiting for the lab to pick it up, and it coagulated. He explained that they were able to run a CBC, but the specific test for the mutation couldn't be done.

So then I asked, "Is there anything else that would cause the liver enzymes to be elevated?"

He said levels that high happen for 1 of 3 reasons: alcohol abuse (nope, that's not it), fatty liver from obesity (nope, that's not it), or cancer of the liver. ☹

Of course, I didn't want to believe that the cancer had metastasized to my liver – that would make it a stage 4 cancer, and would be accompanied by a grim prognosis.

I had trouble wrapping my brain around this new information, especially knowing that my blood sample had been mishandled. I chose not to go down the dark rabbit hole into despair, but instead sat with the information. I asked for a copy of the test results so I could add them to my medical files.

Once I got home, I shared the situation with my husband. We both agreed that it was probably a mistake since the blood had been compromised. I would ask my primary to retest my liver enzymes at my upcoming appointment, and hopefully they would be normal.

QUALITY FAMILY TIME

SEPTEMBER 1, 2018

"It's not selfish to love yourself, take care of yourself, and to make your happiness a priority. It's necessary." ~ Mandy Hale

It was Labor Day weekend, so I decided that we needed a little family bonding time after all of this focus on cancer and healing my body. And what better way to bond than at a water park!!

I knew the kids would love it, so we planned a fun family getaway to the new Great Wolf Lodge! It was only a 45-minute drive away, and they had some amazing deals for their grand opening, so we booked a room and headed to Gurnee!

It's so important to me that we make happy memories with the kids. A cancer journey is hard on everyone involved, but especially children, so any distraction from the seriousness was welcome.

Great Wolf Lodge has an amazing ropes course and rock climbing wall in addition to their waterpark, and we made good use of it! The kids faced their fears on several occasions, and we all got some good exercise!

I'm very happy to say that the folks at the Barnwood Restaurant at the resort were extremely accommodating regarding our dietary restrictions. It is amazing what people are willing to do if you just ask respectfully. They went above and beyond!

It was a wonderful weekend away, and just what the doctor ordered.

MORE VITAMIN C

SEPTEMBER 6, 2018

"I am learning to trust the journey even if I don't understand it" ~ **Rumi**

I returned to the clinic for my next IV infusion, hoping that we'd be able to increase my dosage of vitamin C this time and really start kicking this tumor in the butt!

The nurse entered the room with a larger bag of the glowing yellow liquid and stated that the test results were normal, and we would be doing 50 grams today. Terrific!

I continued to go to this clinic once a week for 50 grams of vitamin C. Unfortunately, they weren't comfortable going any higher than that, which was disappointing. I had read studies of successful treatment of certain cancers using 60 grams, 70 grams, or even 100 grams of vitamin C in each infusion. In my overachieving manner, I wanted to reach the peak to hopefully have the most impact. Alas...

I also had been getting Artemisinin and Ozone Therapy during my IV treatments in Germany and wondered if that could be added to my sessions. The nurse said she was getting trained on both of these treatments in October, and she was excited to 'try it out' on me.

I'll be honest - I had a slightly uncomfortable feeling about continuing at this clinic. They had mishandled my blood draw, they didn't offer the levels or specific treatments (yet) that I was hoping for, and there was the issue of how the doctor handled the delivery of the potentially bad news (elevation of liver enzymes). I began looking for other options...

To learn more about IV vitamin C, check this out: *www.ri-ordanclinic.org/research-study/vitamin-c-research-ivc-protocol*

"In addition to providing ascorbate replenishment, IVC may allow oncologists to exploit some interesting anti-cancer properties, including high dose IVC's ability to induce tumor cell apoptosis, inhibit angiogenesis, and reduce inflammation."

FOLLOW UP ULTRASOUND

SEPTEMBER 10, 2018

"Breathe, darling. This is just a chapter. It's not your whole story." ~ **S. C. Lourie**

A lot had happened since returning from my time at the klinik. Life had been so much more stressful than I ever could have imagined. I did my best to do all of my healing therapies every day and to stick to a clean Vegan diet, but the various matters of family life were weighing heavily on me. I was finding it hard to calm my nerves, and it concerned me.

As directed by my doctor at Marinus, I scheduled a follow up ultrasound to be done 6 weeks after returning from treatments in Germany.

Since we were told that the treatments continue to work for several weeks, we were hopeful that the tumor would be even smaller now. After all, it had already shrunk an additional 0.4 cm after just 3 weeks, and we couldn't have been happier. Was it crazy to think that we could see double the shrinkage after 6 weeks at home? I silently prayed that it would now be under 2 cm...

West accompanied me to Elmhurst Memorial Hospital, where the ultrasound had been ordered. I checked in, and much to my surprise, I was faced with a lot of pressure to get a mammogram in addition to the ultrasound.

I explained that I would no longer be getting mammograms – not now, and not ever.

Not only do I have dense breasts, which makes it difficult to interpret a mammogram and distinguish between cancer and dense tissue (they both appear white), but the enormous pressure put on the breast during a mammogram can damage the delicate breast tissue.

Furthermore, some doctors feel that compressing a tumor between 2 plates using 42 pounds of pressure could rupture the tumor. On top of that, there is the repeated exposure to potentially harmful radiation, which is thought to fuel cancer cell growth. I didn't want any part of it.

Sadly, this would *not* be the last time I would deal with the enormous insistence from Western Medicine that I should follow the standard of care without question. It was even stated that they wouldn't do the ultrasound unless I agreed to do the mammogram.

I did have many mammography images taken in June, and the pain they caused literally brought me to tears. Fortunately, those images were taken within a 6-month window of the scheduled follow up ultrasound, and in light of that, they agreed to do it sans mammogram, solely based on the timing.

Already anxious, I was now irritated and frustrated. I disrobed, put on the paper gown and got up on the cold metal exam table. The technician squirted me with the cold gel and proceeded with the test.

As she measured the mass from every angle, I could see by West's face that it wasn't good news...

When we left Germany, our final ultrasound showed the tumor mass to be 2.4 cm at its largest measurement. On this day, 6 weeks later and after that soul-crushing life event in August, it was now 3.2 cm. It had been consistently shrinking from June 12 (the date of the original diagnostic mammogram and ultrasound), until July 28, when we left the clinic, but suddenly it was going in the wrong direction – the tumor was growing.

This was not at all what I had hoped for, and I was completely devastated. I couldn't hold back the emotions or the fear of what this reality meant for my future, nor could I hold back the tears...

SPINNING

"The soul always knows what to do to heal itself.
The challenge is to silence the mind."
~ Caroline Myss

My head was still spinning from the recent news... I was completely crushed that all of the progress I'd made over the previous 2 months was now lost.

The tumor had shifted directions and was now growing in size at an alarming rate. I had no doubt that this was due to the enormous stress in my life, and my inability to get it under control.

Was it possible that the lab results that the doctor at the IV clinic had so coldly delivered could be accurate, and the cancer had indeed spread to my liver?? The tumor was able to grow nearly a centimeter in 6 short weeks, so clearly something had changed.

I asked my Integrative Medicine doctor to run another

blood test to check my liver enzymes again. She also tested my CA-15-3, which is a cancer marker. CA-15-3 is an antigen that is released into the blood by some kinds of cancer cells, most likely breast cancer cells.

One of the many things I love about Dr. Afridi is that she gets back to me as soon as she gets test results and offers her level-headed opinion.

"Hi Leslie. The labs are back. It does look like the liver enzymes are elevated, and I'm not sure why that is. I suggest we do a liver ultrasound to follow up on this and see what is going on."

Crap... I had convinced myself that the IV clinic had messed up the blood draw and it was all a crazy mistake. I guess that was wishful thinking.

For some reason, none of the doctors in the States had tested my CA-15-3 markers. During treatments in Germany, they were consistently in the normal range (15, give or take a point). Now they were more than double that level, having increased to 33 over that 6-week period,... NOT GOOD.

Something bad was happening inside my body, and I was scared. I no longer felt like I had any control over what was happening. It felt like my body was betraying me.

I shared the breast ultrasound and blood test results with my team of doctors, and they all thought it was a sign that the cancer had spread to my liver... I spiraled into a dark abyss. I had to face the reality that the cancer had most likely spread, which would change the outlook completely. I grew depressed as I pondered my future, and the future of my children.

I scheduled the liver ultrasound for September 18 and started to prepare myself for the rough road ahead.

"Life expectancy for breast cancer with liver metastases without treatment is only four to eight months, but most people seek treatment. With treatment, the 5-year survival rate for people with distant metastases related to breast cancer is 23 percent."

www.verywellhealth.com/breast-cancer-spread-to-the-liver-4135738

FEEL THOSE FEELINGS

"I believe that health is more than merely the
absence of disease.
It is a total state of physical, mental, emotional,
spiritual and social well-being."
~ Dr. Frank Lipman

I gave myself 24 hours to mope and to contemplate the bad news I'd just received. I had tried so hard to stay positive for months, knowing that the mind is a powerful force in healing, but I needed a day to feel sad about this turn of events.

Sometimes you need to allow yourself to FEEL the scary stuff and not just push it down or cover it up with "happy thoughts".

Tampering with the natural flow of emotions puts stress on the mind and body. Some believe that if we don't allow strong emotions to surface, they can manifest in our bodies as disease. Emotional stress from blocked emotions has been linked to many illnesses including autoimmune disorders and cancer.

Perhaps this is why the cancer was able to take hold in my body in the first place... I had a pretty good life, but I had been through some difficult events teeming with complex and overwhelming emotions: my father's near fatal motorcycle accident when I was 8, watching him take his last breaths many years later, enduring years of infertility treatments that never worked, 2 failed adoptions before bringing our baby girl home, betrayals of the heart... when I looked back, I realized how much pain I had experienced that had never truly been unpacked and healed.

NOW FOCUS ON THE GOOD

"If you have enough breath to complain about anything, you have more than enough reason to give thanks about something."
~ Mattie Stepanek

I'd had my little pity party for that day, and now I was ready to focus on GRATITUDE again. After all, there was nothing more I could do at this point except wait to see what showed up on the ultrasound.

I had already determined that, if there was indeed a tumor in my liver as the doctors suspected, I would hop on a plane immediately and head back to Marinus to 'turn this ship back around'.

West was 100% supportive of that plan. Though money was tight (he hadn't had an income since being laid off from his job the previous October), we were determined not to let finances determine my fate. I am still so incredibly grateful for that.

So I turned my focus to all of the amazing people surrounding me with love and positive vibes.

- Grateful for new connections with fellow healers who offer their own version of inspiration. Cancer Thrivers UNITE!

- Grateful for my 'Health Is Our Jam' friends, Janel and Stephanie, who are always willing to try out the latest healing modality with me! Forest Therapy at Morton Arboretum was truly amazing and calming, as was Meditation with Essential Oils (though the rain drove us indoors for that one). Thank you, my friends, for your never-ending positivity and focus on healthy living - you always inspire me to grow and be a better person!

- Grateful for the positive energy and lyrics of Jason Mraz, and the chance to experience it with my dear friend, Jennifer, at Ravinia!

- Grateful for healthy smoothies and walking through nature (and witnessing the release of the Monarchs!), with Bekah.

- Grateful to Jen and Sonny for taking the kids swimming and feeding them dinner - they had a blast! And we made great use of the quiet house.

- Grateful for gabbing over a Vegan snack at LYFE Kitchen with Laurie, who always knows the right thing to say to make me feel better.

- Grateful to Caitlin for the laughter, love and support, the Scenterific candle and the detox soap!

- Grateful to Joy for inviting me to Candlelight Yoga; stretching the body, centering the mind, and calming the spirit along with a sweet friend - how lucky am I?

- Grateful for our 'parents support group' at Wellness House, but especially grateful for the 'kids' support group'. I worry about the big things that they have had to deal with and continue to deal with...

- Grateful for the amazing lavender goodies from the Lavender Farm, a sweet gift from Marti. Sleep cannot elude me now!

- Grateful to my mom, Randy, and Barb for taking the kids on a fun adventure today.

- Grateful for conversation, friendship (spanning almost 40 years!), mutual support, and peppermint tea at Courageous Bakery with Jenny. And I love my beautiful gratitude bracelet! It's a constant reminder to find the silver linings on this journey. Thank you, my sweet friend from long ago. ☺

No matter what you are going through, there is ALWAYS something to be grateful for... and it is humbling. I am so very lucky for the amazing people in my life.

DETOX

"Go inside and listen to your body, because your body will never lie to you.
Your mind will play tricks, but the way you feel in your heart, in your guts, is the truth."
~ Don Miguel Ruiz

I was desperate to detoxify my body, especially my liver, in order to take some of the burden off of my system. Healing cancer is serious business! My body had been working so hard for several months, and it was tired, but I simply couldn't slow down.

Someone suggested that I get regular colonics to help with detoxification, so I did a search for a qualified provider near me.

I discovered a clinic in Westmont and made an appointment for September 16. I wasn't excited about getting this done, but I was willing to try anything once to see if it would help.

The woman spent a lot of time lecturing me on healthy living (preaching to the choir, lady!) and the benefits of regular colonics. She had MANY supplements and products for sale that were displayed around the room. I didn't have a terrific feeling about this, but was trying to keep an open mind.

During the session, she said she witnessed lots of toxins and parasites leaving my body through the tubing. This was amazing... and slightly horrifying. It did give me a boost of confidence that I was indeed ridding my body of this junk, but it was terribly uncomfortable, and I was anxious for it to be over. Eventually, I asked for her to please finish the session as I was tired and very crampy.

Was this experience actually helpful in healing my body? I'm still not sure... it certainly wasn't fun, but I did feel lighter and "cleaned out".

There are conflicting thoughts on colonics. Some feel that it clears out the gunk that gets in the way of the body functioning properly. Some feel that it is a dangerous approach and should be avoided.

In the end (no pun intended ;)), I listened to my body and my instincts. This approach wasn't right for me.

She did have some suggestions of doctors that offered IV treatments, including Ozone Therapy and Artemisinin, so it wasn't a complete loss. I took down the contact information for her two recommendations and added them to my list of possible options for the future.

REALITY CHECK

SEPTEMBER 18, 2018

"I learned that courage was not the absence of fear,
but the triumph over it.
The brave man is not he who does not feel afraid,
but he who conquers that fear."
~ Nelson Mandela

It was the day of the liver ultrasound, and I was incredibly anxious. West told me to stay positive, but the truth was that I needed to prepare myself for potentially bad news.

Going into the previous ultrasound to measure the tumor, I was focusing on positive thoughts, and truly believed we were going to see significant shrinkage. Not being prepared for all possible outcomes was a mistake... hearing that the tumor was growing instead of shrinking was a powerful blow, but going in with the naïve mental state that everything was hunky-dory only set me up for a bigger shock. It was like a slap in the face that I wasn't expecting, and it hit me hard. I didn't want to make that same mistake again.

I was cautiously optimistic, but I also needed to set realistic expectations for myself and prepare for the situation that my team of doctors suspected was going on.

I needed to brace myself for unwelcome news and have a plan in place, so it wouldn't completely rock my world. I needed to be able to move forward with conviction no matter what the ultrasound showed.

And it was vital that I didn't allow fear to take over. When we make decisions from a place of fear, we aren't standing in our power. If we aren't in touch with our intuition, and if we don't tap into that inner voice - perhaps because it's clouded by the incessant rumblings of fear - we cannot hear the whispers telling us what is truly RIGHT for us.

LIVER ULTRASOUND

"Sometimes our lives have to be completely shaken up, changed, and rearranged to relocate us to the place we're meant to be."
~ Adrianne Hemenway

West and I headed to the Edward-Elmhurst Health Center in Hinsdale for the scheduled ultrasound of the liver. The results of this test could completely change the outlook of my future, and I felt the gravity of this day deep in my soul.

Everyone we encountered during this experience was so kind and compassionate, and I am so grateful. My fragile emotions couldn't have handled the typical reaction I had gotten from various staff members at the array of hospitals that I'd been to over the past 3 months. It seems that our overworked healthcare providers usually have limited patience for those of us who don't blindly go along with the advised standard of care, but luckily, today was different. No lectures, no encouragement to follow the "protocol" – just kindness.

It also helped that we weren't sent to a busy and bustling hospital, but instead to a health center, tucked away on a quiet street behind Salt Creek– we seemed to be the only patients there at that time, and it helped ease the nerves coursing through my body.

Honestly, I was ready to know, ready to get answers, and ready to take the next step on this journey – no matter what that step would be.

West and I waited patiently on the welcoming bench set in front of a wide span of windows. The sun was shining outside, and the trees were beginning to turn colors. It was a calming sight.

The technician called us into the room and asked me to do the usual prep for an ultrasound. I took some deep breaths and we began.

She squirted the gel onto my chest and abdomen, but to my surprise, it wasn't ice cold! Oh glory be, what a difference a little heat makes to this experience! I shared my delight with the tech, and she said they installed a warmer on the new ultrasound machine. Thank heavens for small miracles☺

The liver is the largest internal organ in the body. There is a large lobe under the right breast and a smaller lobe under the left breast, much of it hidden behind the ribcage. The tech took many pictures of all areas of my liver, moving in between and around my ribs.

She had a pleasant personality, a welcome quality when dealing with life-altering moments. This was a very serious moment, but in my typical fashion, I tried to lighten the mood with some humor, and she was playing along, which helped buoy my spirits.

After about 20 minutes of scans, I said, "I haven't noticed

her measuring anything... she hasn't stopped to *measure* anything... is it possible there is nothing there to measure?!?"

West had a small hopeful grin on his face, and said, "Nope, she hasn't found anything to measure..." The tech turned to me with a reassuring look and concurred – "Nope, there hasn't been anything for me to measure". Could it be possible??

West and I were both a bit stunned. I got dressed, and we quietly left the room. We had barely taken 2 steps into the hallway when we fell into each other's arms, and the joyful tears began flowing.

I could hardly believe it – there were no tumors appearing in my liver. Hallelujah!!

The tech then approached and handed me a copy of the images. She fully understood that we wanted – no, needed – solid answers, and time was of the essence. Now we could head straight home and send the images off to our team of doctors to get input.

Ultrasound techs aren't allowed to discuss what they see on the scans for liability reasons, but I am so grateful that she was able to give us a little insight to put my mind at ease. We wouldn't have the official results until the radiologist was able to read the images, but for that moment, we celebrated.

AN OVERWHELMED LIVER

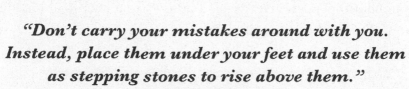

*"Don't carry your mistakes around with you.
Instead, place them under your feet and use them
as stepping stones to rise above them."*
~ Loni Heinen

I felt such relief after learning that there were no tumors in my liver. I could breathe again!

We still needed to figure out why my liver enzymes were so high. Was something overwhelming my liver?

The liver is the main filtration system of the body, and it's responsible for removing chemicals and metabolizing drugs. This is a big job, and it's working almost constantly.

I had a gut feeling that the many supplements I had been taking over the last 3 months were simply too much for my body to handle. I often felt bloated and uncomfortable shortly after taking the numerous pills – perhaps I needed to listen to my body even when I think what I'm doing is good for me.

I've always been a sensitive person – my skin reacts to harsh products, my sense of smell is acute, I get migraines easily from bright light or loud noises, I'm a sympathetic crier. I've long suffered from allergies, struggled with asthma, and was diagnosed with IBS in my 20's. It made sense that my organs were also sensitive and may need a "less is more" approach rather than an "everything that's ever been recommended" approach.

I sent the liver ultrasound results to each of the doctors on my team. Of course, each of them was pleased that no tumors were found, and they all agreed that the supplements might be the cause of the problem.

Here are the thoughts from my Integrative Cancer Specialist:

"Leslie, I wanted to see the ultrasound results first before commenting on the liver tests. There were 2 small gallbladder stones "a.k.a. cholelithiasis", with a normal appearing liver. So in essence, I am not worried about the ultrasound.

When liver enzymes go up, I recommend patients take a break from the supplements to give the liver a break from all that it does on a daily basis, which is to detoxify the blood. Then, recheck the liver enzymes in a week, and see where they are at after that. I don't think the supplements impair the liver, but it's good to stop them to see what happens so we can see if there is indeed an effect.

In the meantime, it looks like you need some "do nothing" time to let your brain decompress from the many activities you're doing. It sounds like balance has gone out of order, and stress is overwhelming. I don't want you to keep juicing and following the diet as strictly if you are feeling dizzy. That's hurting more than helping you. Please spend time enjoying healthy meals with your family, and finding time to devote to good distractions like music, art, spending time with people you love. This will help fill up your tanks because it sounds like they are really depleted with pursuing all of these tests, opinions, health-seeking activities, and so on. The opposite of 'fear' is 'love', and the more you can feel safe, loved, humor, and so on, the less fear will take over."

Wise words, indeed...

WHEN ONE SOLUTION CAUSES ANOTHER PROBLEM

"No matter how much it gets abused, the body can restore balance.
The first rule is to stop interfering with nature."
~ Deepak Chopra

I immediately stopped taking any and all pills in hopes of lowering the liver enzymes and healing whatever was unbalanced. The strange thing is that I hadn't been taking *any* pharmaceuticals. The many pills I was taking were all natural supplements recommended by my doctors. We don't often stop to think about the side effects caused by the pills we take, but many come with their own list of potential problems.

I used to take Advil almost daily because of migraines and back pain. That started causing stomach problems, which in turn led to the doctor suggesting I take Pepcid or Prilosec to deal with the acid reflux (most likely being caused by the large amounts of NSAIDs I was taking).

I also took allergy medicine every morning and often at

night to help me breathe. As the years went by, I needed something stronger and stronger to get the same effect, but the strong
allergy medicine made me feel tired and foggy all day. I wasn't
sure which was worse – feeling like a zombie from the medicine,
or sneezing and itchy eyes...

I also took a daily multi-vitamin because that's what you're
supposed to do. These vitamins usually made my stomach feel
upset.

Several years ago, my migraines began increasing in severity
and I was desperate for a fix. My primary doctor at the time
suggested that I start each day with caffeine, an aspirin, and an
Aleve, and see how that made me feel. Taking even more pills
only made me feel worse in the long run.

She also suggested I see a neurologist to confirm that it
wasn't anything more serious. The neurologist sent me for an
MRI of my brain.

The MRI of my brain was...an interesting experience. They
locked my head in a helmet-like contraption that made me feel
like Hannibal Lecter from *Silence of the Lambs*. I wasn't able to
move or even take a deep breath. They inserted a needle in my
arm (at that point, I didn't understand the dangers of Gadolinium, the contrast agent used in many MRIs), and pushed me
inside of the narrow tube. I only lasted about 20 seconds before
I had trouble breathing and asked to come out. I was shaking
and frazzled from the feeling of being trapped.

The tech said this happened often. She suggested I get a
prescription for Xanax and try again... more pills.

So I did. I took the Xanax, as instructed, and we were able to
get the images. It showed flairs consistent with migraines. Huh...
all that to tell me what I already knew. I officially have
migraines.

The neurologist prescribed some heavy-duty long-term

pharmaceuticals to manage my migraines, and off I went. Surprisingly, one of the side effects of the pills he gave me was, wait for it - SEVERE MIGRAINES!!

Ummm... wait a second... these pills that I'm hoping will stop the incredible pain I've been experiencing might actually make the headaches WORSE!?! Well, that seems backwards. But they are literally manipulating the chemistry in your brain, and apparently, it's a bit of a guessing game.

So I took the pills, like a good patient.

A few hours later, I experienced the most intense and most painful migraine of my life. The kids' giggles made my head nearly explode, and I couldn't handle any daylight or smells. All I could do was crawl under the covers with earplugs and an eye mask, and wait for the torture to pass.

That's when I knew I was done trying to fix every little problem with a pill. I needed to do the tough work and clean up my life! And that's exactly what I did.

I cleaned up my diet, I got myself into a yoga class regularly, I started meditating, and I looked for more joy in my life. I also signed up to become a certified holistic health coach through the Institute for Integrative Nutrition, where I learned so much about how to lead a healthier life.

Often it's a simple solution – simple, but necessarily easy. Most of us don't want to make the necessary changes to *FEEL BETTER*. We want the quick fix, but it takes work and dedication to become our best selves.

And the work is never over – you must stay committed every day. But it's worth it.

FINDING A BALANCE

"You are what you eat. Every 28 days, your skin replaces itself. Your liver, 5 months. Your bones, 10 years. Your body makes these new cells from the food you eat. What you eat literally becomes you. You have a choice in what you're made of."
~ David Wolfe

When I was diagnosed with breast cancer in June, I radically changed my diet because I understood the power of food, and how it can heal our bodies. I was already pretty healthy, having cut out all processed junk, fast foods and fried foods, and cooking most meals at home. But there was still room for improvement, especially when faced with a deadly disease.

So we cut out *all* sugar (even my organic raw honey), all gluten, all animal products, all caffeine, all alcohol. We were serious and 100% committed to healing.

But the truth is that I barely ate anything... I juiced vegetables and maybe ate salads, and made sure everything was organic, but I would get so worried each time I put anything into my mouth.

My mind would race - "Was this an alkalizing vegetable? Did this fruit have anti-angiogenic properties? Was there too much natural sugar in the pineapple that I so enjoyed? Was this bite going to fuel the cancer??" It was a constant struggle.

I had lost nearly 30 pounds in those first 3 months, and I wasn't heavy in the first place. At my lowest weight, I was 113 pounds on a 5 foot 9 inch frame. My energy was non-existent – I had trouble just walking up the stairs or washing my hair, at times. Something needed to change.

West and I agreed that I needed more calories, and felt that it would be smart to incorporate some carbs beyond brown rice and quinoa (I wasn't a huge fan of either, though I know they are good whole grain choices).

We began eating gluten-free pasta with homemade tomato sauce and homemade baked tortilla chips with hummus on occasion. My weight stabilized and my energy improved.

DR. WEBER'S INPUT

OCTOBER 10, 2018

"Your body has the capacity of self healing.
What you have to do is allow it, to authorize it to
heal." ~ Thich Nhat Hanh

Dr. Weber, my doctor at the clinic in Germany, received the results from the ultrasound of my liver and said he didn't think the elevated enzymes were a sign of metastases. He agreed that the many supplements I'd been taking were likely to blame, and even mentioned that the supplements could cause the CA15-3 levels to rise, which I hadn't heard before.

He also concurred that a CT scan wasn't our next step. It gave me some relief to have an MD agreeing that it's best to avoid additional toxic testing at this point.

It's such a guessing game, no matter what path you're taking...

THE TUMOR IS A SYMPTOM

SEPTEMBER 21, 2018

"You are always on your path. The obstacles aren't put there to stop you, they are there to strengthen your desire." ~ **Carol CC Miller**

The recent happenings in the growth of the tumor, the rise in my cancer markers, and the liver scare made me feel a bit shaken and questioning elements of my path.

I am part of several cancer support groups, many focused on natural healing, and it is often said that you have to change things up every so often to "keep cancer on its toes". Even my oncologist said it, and followed it by saying this also happens with chemo – they often have to switch medicines because it stops working after a few months.

The cancer gets "smart" and finds a way to keep proliferating. It is said that cancer will do anything to keep on living, even if it ends up killing its host and thus creating its own demise. Stupid cancer...

I knew that I needed to deal with the stressful situation at home that was still weighing on me, though less intensely than it did at first. Stress was clearly playing a large role in the reversal of my progress.

And perhaps I needed to reconsider having this thing removed... I was hoping that, with all of my efforts, I would be able to eliminate the tumor using alternative medicine, but it was no longer shrinking. This sucker was stubborn.

The truth is - the tumor was just a symptom of a systemic problem. Something was wrong with my immune system that allowed this mass to grow out of control. Removing it would only be a temporary solution, a band-aid of sorts, and wouldn't address the larger issues. If I didn't fix the root problem, it would simply grow back, as it does with so many people, regardless of whether they do conventional treatment or not.

Yet maybe, just maybe, I needed a little help.

All of my efforts have been so ultra-focused on the tumor. Maybe if it wasn't there, it would take a load off of my immune system and allow my body to heal any other areas that might need attention, so this didn't become a bigger problem.

I decided I'd do some more research on the benefits and risks involved in a lumpectomy (also called a partial mastectomy). Then I made an appointment with my surgeon to discuss some questions that were on my mind.

As always, he was calm, confident and willing to listen – and more importantly, willing to answer all of my questions.

I left his office with more clarity, as well as more confidence that he would indeed be my surgeon if I decided to take this step. Though I still wasn't ready for something so drastic. It just didn't feel like it was time.

Instead, West and I discussed going back to Marinus in Germany for another 3 weeks of treatments. We reached out to the doctor there and waited for his reply.

THINGS WEREN'T FEELING RIGHT

SEPTEMBER 25, 2018

"Be strong enough to stand alone, smart enough to know when you need help, and brave enough to ask for it." ~ Mark Amend

I reached out to one of the recommendations that I had gotten for clinics that offer high-dose vitamin C infusions as well as other therapies. The prices were manageable, and they offered more than just the vitamin C – I could also get Ozone Therapy and Artemisinin IVs, both of which had been part of my treatment in Germany. So I made my first appointment.

This doctor worked out of a rented room at a clinic in Lisle. I arrived at the address I had been given, but this doctor wasn't listed on the directory. I called the nurse who had scheduled my appointment, but there was no answer. I sat in the lobby for 20 minutes before she called me back and told me where to go. Not a great start...

I met with Dr. J. in a side office. He was a young muscle-packed man with long blonde hair pulled back into a bun on top of his head. I asked if he would be willing to administer 60 grams of vitamin C, to which he responded, "Why not do 75 grams!" Hmmm... he was strangely enthusiastic.

I did find it strange that he didn't require any sort of blood test before starting high doses, nor was he particularly interested in seeing my blood test results from the first IV clinic. He also didn't hesitate to combine all 3 therapies into one treatment. Marinus had always spread them out over the week so my body wasn't overwhelmed.

He was alarmingly cavalier, but I was desperate to get any and all natural treatments that I could find to recreate my protocol in Germany.

I was then led into a common sitting area that wasn't particularly clean or welcoming. He set up my IV, and then administered the Ozone Therapy followed by Artemisinin. As soon as the blood started leaving my body, I felt a little bit woozy.

Once those treatments were completed, he arrived with a large bag filled with a glowing yellow liquid – the 75 grams of vitamin C. I had seen this at the previous clinic, but they had always kept it covered with a dark shield. I had been told that vitamin C is sensitive to light and oxygen in the atmosphere, so it needed to be protected. When I asked Dr. J. why he didn't have his vitamin C bags covered, he said it wasn't necessary. Hmmm...

As the drops slowly entered the needle in my arm, I began to feel incredibly thirsty. That is a normal reaction to high doses of vitamin C, so I wasn't too worried. However, the longer the infusion went on, the more I began to feel faint. I was chatting with an old friend of mine on the phone and was suddenly having trouble thinking straight or forming sentences. I was getting very tired, and said I had to hang up and find the doctor.

The nurse finally walked by, and I stopped her to say that I wasn't feeling very well. She asked if I wanted something from their basket of snacks, but the options were all full of sugar, and I wasn't about to undo any good I had created by eating junk. Note to self: bring your own healthy snacks.

She asked the doctor to come by and check on me. When he finally appeared, he said it was probably nothing to worry about, but perhaps we should stop the drip a little early. He suggested I bring carb-heavy food along next time, so I don't have a similar reaction (I had only eaten a salad during the 4-hour infusion), and sent me on my way.

I got into the car and called West via Bluetooth, telling him about the experience. About 10 minutes into the drive, a crushing headache set in. The symptoms progressively got worse on the trip home, and West was sounding worried. I kept telling him that I could make it, but then a deep exhaustion suddenly came over me - I had trouble completing my sentences or holding my head up.

I was around the corner from my home by this point, so I kept going - in hindsight, I should have pulled over immediately and asked him to come and get me. I barely made it home and immediately collapsed on the couch. I woke up an hour later with West standing over me, begging me to eat something.

I'm still surprised that the doctor sent me home when I started having signs of trouble... he was confident that it wouldn't be a problem in the future if I made sure to eat lots of carbs before and during the treatment.

UPDATING THE GROUP

SEPTEMBER 26, 2018

"Sometimes I just want someone to hug me and say, I know it's hard. Here's a chocolate and 6 million dollars." **~ Author Unknown**

We decided that we should update our support team and finally let them know what had been happening... I didn't want to worry anyone, but now that I had some time to process things, I wanted to share details and keep everyone in the loop.

West's post to the private FB group:

"Two-months since our return from Germany Update

We know that many of you have been wondering what our last update meant (alluding to good and bad news) and probably have been trying to read between the lines. First, I want to say thank you for not hounding us for the details. We have been working through all of the emotions and options in front of us for the last couple of weeks and are finally ready to share the details.

On the good side, the ultrasound we had a couple of weeks

back showed that the suspicious area in her left breast had shrunk by 50% and is more than likely nothing at all to worry about. We will keep a watchful eye on it over the next year. They also checked her lymph nodes, and they all seem to be clear. More good news.

However, the cancerous tumor in the right breast was measured at 3.2 cm, which is bigger than when we left Germany. Not the largest measurement we've seen thus far (the original ultrasound showed it to be 3.6 cm), but certainly not the news we were hoping for.

It took us a while and a consultation with a surgeon to wrap our heads around it, but we believe it could be one of two scenarios:

1. Either the tumor really has never changed, it's always been around 3 cm give or take, and this is a measurement "margin of error" issue (which, on the bright side, means that this aggressive and invasive tumor has been stable for 3 months!).
2. Or our transition back from Germany and all of the good progress we made there was undone by a pretty stressful situation back home. We have learned that cancer feeds off of stress hormones, and tumor growth has a 60% correlation with the amount of stress a person is experiencing.

In addition, Leslie has had two blood tests since we have been back. All prior blood tests have always been in normal ranges – they never even show any cancer markers. These recent tests showed that her liver enzymes were high. Potential causes of high liver enzymes are alcohol abuse, obesity, supplements, and cancer metastasis. Our minds went immediately to the concern that the cancer had spread to her liver.

After several very terrifying days while waiting for the ultrasound, we are glad to report that her liver is clear and that all of her doctors believe it is due to the myriad of supplements she has been taking. She has stopped taking them and will be having another blood test tomorrow to see if the levels come back down into the normal range.

As I mentioned above, we had a visit with Dr. Winchester, who is our surgeon of choice if we decide to go down that path. During the visit, he seemed surprised that the tumor was the same size as when we had seen him 3 months ago. I take that as an encouraging sign that what we have been doing has, at a minimum, stopped it from growing. For now, we're going to continue to monitor the growth before taking any further steps toward surgery since it's a big decision and there's no turning back once you go down that road.

Now that we have caught you up on the past, we wanted to give everyone an update on our future plans that continue to evolve as we learn more. Leslie has found some local places to get many of the treatments that she was having in Germany, with the exception of Hyperthermia. She has been getting high dose Vitamin C/Artemisinin/Ozone therapy/Vitamin B infusions, doing daily dry skin brushing and meditation in the Infrared Sauna, and found a place to do BioMat a few times a week, along with all of the other things we have been doing since we have been back.

In addition, we are planning on heading back to Germany with the kids during the Thanksgiving break. Leslie will stay on for another week or two after we leave, so that she can continue her treatments like the last time. The kids and I will come home so they don't miss school (much to their chagrin).

We apologize that we haven't shared many of these tidbits with all of you before now, but we really needed to work through our thoughts and feelings. As always, we ask that you continue to send all the positive thoughts and prayers her way! I can't tell you how much it helps her keep the positive attitude she needs.

We are trying to get her back to being a human with a disease as opposed to a disease that is human on occasion. Therefore, I have a request (but please don't tell her I said this!). I was hoping that some of you crazy people out there would be willing to take her out to have some fun! Anything that can just take her mind off of the cancer and/or make her laugh would be awesome. You don't have to avoid the subject, but find something that will draw her focus away for a while. Take her to a movie, an art class, concert, or roller skating (she will kill me for suggesting that one). She isn't in the planning mode at this point, so, bring her some ideas and ask her for some free dates and see what magic can happen – oh you could take her to a magic show!!!!"

A FAMILY AFFAIR

*"When you cannot control the situation, challenge
yourself to control how you respond to the
situation. This is where your power lies."*
~ Author Unknown

My niece was getting married on a beach in Florida at the end
of September, and I was determined not to let cancer keep me
from an important family event. So I made arrangements to fly
down there and do my best to be a part of the festivities.

I flew by myself to Destin, picked up my rental car at the
airport, and drove about an hour and a half to the two-bedroom
condo I had rented by the beach. It was a long drive alone in the
rain, and I was nervous about getting lost in a strange place. I
was so sensitive to stressors since my diagnosis, but I tried not to
let it overwhelm me.

Along the way, I found a Whole Foods with a juice bar, so I
grabbed a healthy green juice and picked up a bunch of
groceries to fill the fridge.

The condo was very spacious and had an extra bedroom, so I invited my mom to stay with me and keep me company. It was a great opportunity for us to spend quality time together, and for that I am grateful.

My mom was willing to explore the area with me a bit, and we stumbled upon a place called Clean Juice only a few minutes away from the condo. They juiced fresh to order, which can be hard to find. My mom agreed to accompany me each morning to get a healthy start to our day. ☺

My post to the private group on September 30:

"Today's delicious breakfast with my mama - Beet juice and steel-cut oats with fresh fruit and coconut.

So grateful to have found this place! Though it's shocking to me how so many supposedly healthy things in this country have added sugar - even at a clean juice bar. The almond butter had added sugar, the vanilla had added sugar, the protein powder had added sugar, the gluten-free bread had added sugar... I had to skip all of those things. I'm learning that you MUST ask them to read the label if you truly want to know what's in your food (which thankfully they were willing to do - and they were also surprised by what they learned)."

It was wonderful to spend time with my family, but I did find myself getting tired very easily. I made sure to take time each day to rest. But I am grateful that I was able to be there to witness the gorgeous ceremony, and party with the entire clan afterwards to celebrate Chelsea and Scott.

A WONDERFUL NEW ADDITION TO MY TEAM

OCTOBER 2, 2018

"If you believe it will work out, you'll see opportunities.
If you believe it won't, you will see obstacles."
~Wayne Dyer

A friend of mine (a fellow Cancer Thriver) told me about an Integrative Oncologist nearby. That's what had been missing from my team of doctors – a specialist who understood cancer, but also understood alternative approaches.

I made an appointment to meet with Dr. L. at Amita Cancer Center in Hinsdale. She reviewed my files and then asked what I was looking for from her. "Are you looking for treatment, or do you want me to simply monitor you?" I explained that I wasn't interested in chemotherapy or radiation, but was hoping for her guidance more than anything, and thankfully, she was willing to play that role in my journey.

She had blood drawn and checked my CA-15-3 levels.

Sadly, they had more than doubled since we left Germany, 9 weeks prior. Oh dear...

She also checked my liver enzymes, and I was thrilled to learn that they were back to normal!! She thought it was one of the mushroom supplements or the Astragalus that overwhelmed my liver and caused the enzymes to rise.

My post to the private FB group:

"Happy to report that my liver enzymes have returned to normal! Doctors have all concluded that it was one or more of the supplements that I have been taking, and have narrowed it down to 3 possible suspects that were all added since my return from Germany (I stopped taking everything for the last 2 weeks). I can either add them back in one by one and get follow up blood tests, or just cut those 3 out of my protocol. (2 of the 3 suspects were mushroom supplements! The evil fungus!!) Guess what my choice is?!? Yep...no more mushrooms for me!

I had a consult with a new Integrative Oncologist this afternoon, and when we discussed the liver issues, she offered to immediately have blood drawn and results would be back in 15 minutes! WOW! I had blood drawn at a lab last week to check the liver and discovered today that they ran the wrong tests ☹ (the *incorrect* test has reconfirmed that my kidneys are functioning well, and my calcium and potassium levels are still good ;)), so this was so fortuitous. I am SO grateful for the peace of mind!!

This oncologist is willing to be my cancer guide on this journey and help with monitoring as I travel along this holistic path. She trained under Dr. Weil and firmly believes that food is medicine, and that diet and lifestyle play a significant role in our health. I'm hoping that having her on my team of doctors will help alleviate my feelings of 'floating in the ocean' without guidance on this very scary journey. And she seemed willing to order ultrasounds without forcing mammograms! YES!!

She stated that medical doctors are only given 15 minutes of nutrition education, so we can't blame them for not educating their patients, which is why she chose to study further with Dr. Weil. She admitted that she believes in traditional treatments, but was willing to listen to my beliefs and support me. She still came on strong at times and put some fear-based pressure on me, but I stayed true to my gut and my path.

She referenced the scientific research and how it is lacking for alternative approaches, but admitted that there will likely never be funding for large trials on these approaches since you can't put a patent on food and lifestyle changes. Which means there is no money to be made from this path, therefore, we'll never have solid evidence. Sad but true..."

TRIPLE NEGATIVE IS TRICKY

"If you're not getting the answers you want or need, do your own due diligence and conduct your own research to find the answers you are looking for." ~
DR. Nasha Winters

I shared an article on my private FB page regarding the metabolic profiling of triple negative breast cancer. It was encouraging to me that our choices can indeed make a significant difference.

"So...triple negative breast cancer (TNBC) is particularly tricky because it isn't hormone driven, thus every doctor I consulted with did the obligatory 'head tilt' of sympathy, knowing full well there were no targeted therapies for this type of cancer.

However, I've recently been encouraged by research and discussions that TNBC has a metabolic connection, which may explain why our radical diet change (and other lifestyle changes) has halted the growth of this highly aggressive cancer.

I read that an increase in abdominal fat showed an increased incidence of TNBC. This is interesting because I've always carried my extra weight across my belly - even now with the extreme weight loss, I'm still holding on to the excess in that area (Why?!? My skinny legs have gotten skinnier, but could I finally have a flat belly??? NO!! It's absolutely maddening...)

But there's hope...

Another study stated, "performing exercise equivalent to walking 30 minutes six days per week and consuming more than 5 daily servings of fruits and vegetables decreased mortality by 46%" (who wants to take a walk with me?) And being Vegan and juicing so much, we easily get 15-20 servings of fruits/veggies daily!

It also stated "alcohol consumption also appears to moderate recurrence and mortality... consumption of 3 to 4 alcoholic drinks or more per week was associated with a 35% increased risk of breast cancer recurrence and 51% increased risk of death due to breast cancer". Again, this solidifies our stance to NOT have that glass of wine with dinner!

These insights strengthen my resolve that this is a change for LIFE (not just while the tumor is apparent) in order to increase my chances of never having a recurrence in the future and living to the ripe old age of 104 (my grandmother's age).

As always, thank you for your support as we navigate this journey. It's scary because so much is unknown when it comes to cancer, but the love and positive vibes from all of you keep me STRONG."

IS ALCOHOL HARMING OUR HEALTH?

*"The doctor of the future will no longer treat the human frame with drugs,
but rather will cure and prevent disease with nutrition."* ~ **Thomas Edison**

I posted an article about the deleterious effects of alcohol on our bodies. A friend then posted a contradictory article in the comments of my post that suggested it wasn't all that bad.

If you want to believe something is good for you, inevitably you can find an article or a study that supports it, whether it be chocolate, coffee, or alcohol. Back in the day, it was even believed that smoking was a healthy choice, or at the very least, wasn't harmful to our health. Cigarettes were even 'doctor recommended'. Clearly, things have changed.

Many producers of these products will fund a study specifically designed to find the health benefits so they can highlight that positive attribute. That marketing piece of gold will help them sell tons of products. And let's be honest – who wouldn't like to believe that your daily indulgence of chocolate, your evening glass of wine, or your morning coffee is actually supporting your health!

We can find something 'good' in almost everything that has 'bad' to it. However, the more I learn and the more I'm truly honest with myself (and not blinded by what I *want* to believe), the more I see that alcohol is toxic to the body. And it is essential that I reduce the toxins that I put into my body, especially now.

It is actually an important consideration for all of us. One glass of wine, one cigarette, one piece of fried chicken won't kill us... right away. It is a culmination of all of our choices over our entire life that determines our true health.

The effects are cumulative, which is exactly why we notice the effects of our toxic choices more and more as we get older - our habits and choices are literally catching up with us.

Nutritional science changes often, which makes it incredibly difficult to know what is the "truth". But we don't need a scientist or the government to tell us that eating REAL food that's as close to its natural state as possible is the smartest way to eat for a healthy and long life. What we put into our bodies on a daily basis really does make a difference – every single bite.

THINK DIRTY

"The average woman puts 515 synthetic chemicals on her body every day without knowing, and 60 percent of what we put onto our skin is absorbed into our bodies." ~ **HuffPost**

I started looking around for other ways to 'clean' up my life and reduce the toxic load on my body. I was shocked at how many things I hadn't considered before!

At every turn, I discovered another element that may be contributing to my struggle to heal my body. I needed to make some changes.

My sweet niece, Chelsea, suggested this app to help:

"I was listening to a podcast the other day and heard about a new app called 'Think Dirty' and thought of you. It provides you a rating 0-10 (10 being the most toxic) for the toxicity of any cosmetic or personal care products and gives you detailed info on the different ingredients. I think it might be helpful for you if you are looking at that aspect to cleanse as well! It is free!"

IF AT FIRST YOU DON'T SUCCEED...

OCTOBER 5, 2018

"Embrace the struggle and let it make you stronger.
It won't last forever." ~ **Tony Gaskins**

I called Dr. J. to make an appointment for my 2nd IV infusion. I would make sure that I brought plenty of carbs along in hopes of avoiding the dreaded reactions!

During our call, he mentioned that he also rents an office space in Hinsdale, so I decided to try this alternate location to see if it was cleaner and more welcoming. And indeed it was.

West insisted on going with me to this next session to make sure I got home safely if I did have adverse reactions again. I felt much more secure having him along and was glad to have him in the driver's seat. Even without the awful reactions, these kinds of infusions often result in fatigue, so I was happy to not be driving.

Dr. J. took me into a room, and I made myself comfortable on a treatment bed. Typically these infusions are administered while the patient is sitting, but because of my previous reaction, he thought it would be helpful to have me lying down.

West had packed numerous snacks including popcorn, potatoes and veggies, and encouraged me to eat periodically throughout the various treatments. We also brought along a gallon of water, and I drank the entire thing during the 4-hour infusion.

We began with the Ozone Therapy followed by the Artemisinin. As always, I was slightly woozy after the 50 ml of blood was removed, but it was bearable.

Then Dr. J. appeared with the giant vitamin C bag (not protected... grrr...), stating that he had removed the Magnesium. He suspected that the Magnesium was causing the sleepiness and was certain this would alleviate any problems. Alas...

As the glowing yellow liquid containing 75 grams of vitamin C slowly dripped into my veins, I began to get a crushing headache. I had to go to the bathroom several times, as you can imagine, and each time I got up from the table, the effects were worse. It got to the point that I couldn't even sit up without assistance. There was no way I would have been able to drive myself home safely.

Dr. J. practically disappeared during this stretch, so I was especially grateful to have West there to track him down when I wasn't feeling well. Dr. J. said he didn't understand why I was still having these reactions – he hadn't seen this in any other patient to this extent. What can I tell you... I'm more sensitive than most!

West drove me home and I passed out on the couch for an hour.

Clearly, removing the Magnesium made no difference, nor did the copious amounts of water and carb-laden food. Dr. J.

thought maybe if we did the various infusions in a different order, perhaps it would make a difference.

I was willing to suffer through these side effects in the name of healing. I'm sure it was nothing compared to the side effects of chemotherapy, so I just had to grin and bear it.

I made an appointment for October 12 to try one more time, but in a different order...I really did want to do whatever alternatives I could find to stop this tumor from growing, even if it meant I was out of commission for an entire day every week.

THE DENTAL CONNECTION

*"Trust your intuition. You don't need to explain or
justify your feelings to anyone,
just trust your own inner guidance, it knows best."*
~ Author Unknown

I had been reading about the dangers of amalgam fillings and
had been considering having my one silver filling removed from
my mouth.

Most dentists have switched to composite resin fillings
instead of using amalgam, perhaps because of the concerns over
the mercury vapors that can be released into the body each time
you chew or brush your teeth. When there are other options,
why take the risk?

While researching, I came across an article that talked about
the connection between the particular tooth that contained the
mercury filling in my own mouth and the various areas of the
body. It's called the Acupuncture Meridian System. My filling
was in the 4th tooth from the center to the right side of my body

– and it turns out this tooth is directly connected to your breast tissue in this system. Huh...

As fate would have it, there was a woman in the chair next to me at one of my IV infusions at the first clinic – the only time there was another person in the room with me – who had her amalgam fillings removed. We spent several hours talking about the research and the current thinking. It was fascinating to speak with her and hear about her experience firsthand. I believe our paths crossed for a reason.

After careful consideration and discussions with my dentist, I decided it would be prudent to indeed have it removed and reduce the toxins potentially being leached into my body.

Every step in the right direction was getting me closer to healing.

Oct 8, 2018 – My dentist removed my mercury filling

"Mercury toxicity impacts every system in your body in the following ways:

1. It poisons your endocrine system by focusing on the thyroid and adrenal glands in particular;
2. It impacts your mental and emotional health because it is a neuro-toxin;
3. It affects your digestive system because it mixes with food and goes down the digestive tract;
4. It can cause inflammation through chronic exposure (remember that inflammation is the underlying cause of many dis-eases, including cancer);
5. It greatly impacts your immune system through increasing the presence of ANA antibodies in the bloodstream, among other things."

www.breastcancerconqueror.com

THE CANNABIS OPTION

"You don't always need a plan. Sometimes you just need to breathe, trust, let go, and see what happens." ~ **Mandy Hale**

Ninety days after submitting the application for my medical cannabis card, the card finally arrived in our mailbox.

We had been reading about the Rick Simpson Protocol, or RSO (Rick Simpson Oil). Rick was a man who treated his cancer successfully by creating a full spectrum cannabis extract with incredibly high levels of THC (Tetrahydrocannabinol) and ingesting it daily. THC is the main psychoactive compound found in cannabis.

THC has been shown to kill cancer cells in laboratory studies, so this was interesting to me. We had heard many stories of healing with nothing but RSO, so it made sense to consider adding it to my bag of healing options.

"Cannabinoid therapies are particularly promising for tumor-producing cancers given that 'no overtly cannabis-resistant tumors have been described so far,' according to the Spanish researchers.

Considering how different cancer subtypes are, and the fact that the viability of non-transformed cells (i.e. healthy cells) is not affected by cannabinoids at the concentrations they kill tumor cells, it is tempting to speculate that these compounds tackle essential, as yet unidentified, cellular functions that all cancer cells share, and that are absent in their non-cancerous counterparts.

Triple-negative, the breast cancer subtype with the worst prognosis, does not generally respond well to chemotherapy. But the Spanish group found that THC and THC-rich cannabis oil both offer some hope in improving treatment outcomes for this highly aggressive cancer."

www.projectcbd.org/medicine/thc-versus-breast-cancer

With the help of my Integrative Cancer Specialist, I discovered that *Mindful,* a recommended Medical Marijuana Dispensary, was only minutes from my home. I called and made an appointment to meet with the owner and discuss my options.

When we arrived, I was surprised to see a lovely space, well organized and clean. I guess I was expecting it to be dark and dirty, and maybe a bit shady or inappropriate, but the dispensary didn't have that feeling at all.

We met the owner, and he talked us through the myriad of choices – and man, were there a LOT of choices!

He explained the health benefits such as pain relief, anxiety relief, appetite stimulation, mood management, and sleep support. He also explained the differences between CBD (Cannabidiol) and THC (Tetrahydrocannabinol), the biggest difference being that THC creates psychoactive effects often referred to as a "high".

I specifically asked him about RSO. He was very familiar

with it and had heard stories of its healing powers. However, he warned me that the amounts of THC taken in this protocol were incredibly high, and I would need to take it several times a day. He said I should expect to be incapable of handling most responsibilities for 3-6 months while taking RSO. Ummmm... what!?!

That simply wasn't an option for me while raising two young children and maintaining an acting career. I needed to be able to care for my kids and participate in family activities. Furthermore, I would need to drive myself downtown for bookings and be able to perform with energy and focus.

The RSO approach was taken off the table, at least for now. I just couldn't commit to being out of commission in all aspects for that long.

Instead, we were given pills, some with CBD only, and some with both CBD and THC. The owner also suggested a cream to use in the evenings that would help me sleep through the night that contained essential oils as well as larger amounts of THC.

I used the cream directly on my tumor, and it did help me sleep a bit better. I was also hopeful that it was indeed having an effect on the cancer cells themselves.

THREE STRIKES YOU'RE OUT

OCTOBER 12, 2018

*"Love yourself enough to set boundaries. Your time and energy are precious. You get to choose how you use it. You teach people how to treat you by deciding what you will and won't accept." ~ **Anna Taylor***

I went for my 3rd session of IV infusions with Dr. J. – 75 grams of vitamin C, Ozone Therapy, and Artemisinin.

Unfortunately, I still had the same terrible reactions – the crushing headache, the extreme fatigue. Dr. J didn't understand why this was happening to me and had run out of suggestions.

There was something about this whole situation that just didn't feel right... I had lost all confidence in Dr. J. and my intuition was telling me that this wasn't the place for me. I still believed in the treatments, but I needed to start the hunt again for a clinic that I trusted...

TO RETREAT OR NOT TO RETREAT

*"Good friends help you find important things when you have lost them… things like your smile, your hope and your courage." ~ **Author Unknown***

When I was diagnosed in June, I decided that it was necessary to cancel my upcoming wellness retreats scheduled for the fall. I simply wouldn't have the time or energy to lead others in wellness when I needed to focus on strengthening my own body and healing this cancer.

The local retreat at Eaglewood Resort was scheduled for August. My contact there was incredibly understanding of my situation, and we agreed to touch base in a year to see if we could reschedule the retreat for late 2019. I made lots of calls to presenters and attendees and refunded money, but I am certain it was the right decision for me.

The destination retreat scheduled for Oct 17 – 21 at Red Mountain Resort in Utah was a different story… they agreed to cancel the retreat, but refused to refund my $500 deposit.

I asked if they would be willing to put that money towards a stay for myself – after all, it is an amazing place, and being in the mountains is always rejuvenating and healing to the soul. I could really use a getaway focused on healing.

They said they would allow me to put the $500 towards a 5-day package, but it had to be during the dates already booked. So I reached out to a dear friend and asked if she might consider going with me, and thankfully she agreed. A wonderful excuse to spend some quality time together.

My post to the private FB group:

"A fabulous weekend in nature with my dear friend, Jen. So very thankful for this time with you, and grateful that you took time out of your busy life to spend it with me! Lots of adventures (hiking, yoga, getting into a hammock!!), and self-care (detoxification spa package including skin brushing, mud wraps, Thai massage), and most importantly, lots and lots of friendship!! I also have to give her a huge shout out for being VEGAN all weekend, in solidarity!! BRAVO my friend! You are so impressive and such an incredible friend."

WHERE DID MY STAMINA GO?

During the weekend in Utah, we had at least one hike in the red rocks scheduled for each day, and sometimes two in a day. On our first morning at the resort, we set out at 8:30 am on a guided two-hour hike through Snow Canyon. I was excited to get out into nature!

But after about an hour, I realized that I had reached my peak of exertion and was feeling worn out. Unfortunately, we were only halfway through the planned hike, and there were many other people on this excursion with us, so there was no turning back. I toughed it out, but it took everything in me to keep up with the group through to the end.

With the dramatic weight loss and the amount of stress that I'd been dealing with, my body wasn't capable of doing what it could do even a handful of months prior. I went in thinking I was just as strong as ever, but the truth was that I was different, and I needed to be gentle with myself.

We had what was sure to be an amazing hike through the lava tubes scheduled for that same afternoon, but I knew in my gut that I would be pushing myself too far if I did another hike that same day. It was essential to re-evaluate my schedule and fit in more rest and down time.

I asked Jen to go on the hike without me – I didn't want her to miss out on a spectacular experience! I also said I would only be doing one of the hikes the following day, but I encouraged her to do the morning Puppy Hike without me. I would spend some time alone while she was gone, and save my strength for the Mindful Sunset Hike that evening. That hike turned out to be my favorite of all of the hikes we did that weekend, and I'm so glad I had the energy to do it.

Jen had an amazing time hiking with the dogs. I decided to spend my time alone watching Kris Carr's *Healing Cancer Summit* and doing some emotional work. And I'm so glad I did... there was one segment of the summit that touched me deeply. And being alone in my hotel room allowed me to feel my emotions completely, something that I don't often have the 'space' to do with others around. I surprised myself by allowing the overwhelming feelings to surface, and I wept uncontrollably. The emotions came pouring out. It was cathartic and healing, and though it was hard to choose being alone rather than being out in the mountains with my friend, I knew I had made a healthy decision for myself in that moment.

I learned that I needed to listen to my body and not push it beyond its current limits. That is a valuable lesson for all of us. I learned that finding the space to get truly quiet and deal with the fear and the doubt going on inside was necessary.

THERMOGRAPHY

"Why worry? If you've done the very best you can,
worrying won't make it any better."
~ Walt Disney

There are moments on this journey when your mind races and you wonder what is truly happening inside your body – the things you can't see or feel.

I knew that I didn't want to do any testing that could potentially be harmful such as mammograms or CT scans, but not knowing how things were progressing was weighing heavy on me. It had been many weeks since my last ultrasound, and we still didn't know if we had stopped the growth of this invasive tumor.

I decided that I wanted to get a thermography, as it was a non-toxic way to monitor any progress. Unfortunately, my insurance didn't cover this test, but it was worth the $250 out of pocket to be able to keep track of any changes happening on this journey.

I found a doctor near me who was trained in holistic medicine and believed in my path, so I scheduled an appointment for October 25 to have thermography images taken of my entire chest as well as my lymph nodes.

"The primary way that thermal imaging works is by detecting temperature variations related to blood flow and demonstrating abnormal patterns associated with the progression of tumors. When the body is viewed through a thermal imaging camera, warm areas stand out against cooler areas, and changes in patterns can be tracked over time. Because cancer cells are growing and multiplying very fast, blood flow and metabolism are higher in the areas near a growing tumor, which means skin temperature near these locations increases. Thermography is not invasive, is low-cost, and does not require use of radiation."

www.draxe.com/thermography

At the doctor's request, I arrived early to acclimate my body to the temperature of the room. The doctor did the scan, and sent them away to be analyzed. When I called to follow up on the results, she told me that something had gone wrong with the test, and we'd have to do it again... hmmmm...

So I returned to the doctor's office on November 5 for a repeat thermography, and we waited for the results.

Strangely, the report said that the test showed NO signs of cancer in either breast. How can that be?? As far as I knew, I had a large active tumor on my right side... the doctor couldn't explain it.

Perhaps everything I'd done had eliminated any blood vessels to the tumor?!? Had our anti-angiogenesis approach indeed had an effect? Perhaps all of our efforts had made this tumor inactive and thus, it wasn't creating any heat...

Did I dare believe that??

MOVING FORWARD

OCTOBER 30, 2018

"Don't forget that healing takes time. The body is a complicated, miraculous system. Give yourself the gift of time and patience and each body processes change in its own time." ~ Yancy Lael

My post to the private FB group:

"Hi all! I wanted to post an update for anyone following along on this journey.

First, we have booked our flights to return to Marinus am Stein in Germany for 3 more weeks of holistic cancer treatments! West and the kids will be joining me for the first week. YAY!

We'll leave after school on Friday November 16 and land in Amsterdam on Saturday morning to be tourists for the weekend. We're going to take the kids to Zaanse Schans to climb inside a windmill, have custom wooden shoes made for each of them, and learn how fresh cheese is made! Then, we'll take a train up to Hoorn so I can show them where I lived and started my theatre company. On Sunday, we'll explore the amazing city of Amsterdam on a canal cruise and then by foot!

We'll fly into Munich early Monday morning, and I'll begin my 2nd round of holistic treatments. West and the kids will fly home the following Sunday, and I'll stay an additional 2 weeks to finish treatments. I will return to Chicago December 7, hopefully with a much smaller tumor!

In the meantime, my new Integrative Oncologist, Dr. L., has ordered a follow up ultrasound for November 7, which will be the first measurement in over 8 weeks, so we're anxious to get the results! She will also test my cancer markers to compare to the previous blood test, which was a little high. We will meet with her on November 12 to discuss the findings.

It was important to her (and to us) to have measurements done in the States just before heading to Germany – it will allow us to compare the tests from the 2 countries and truly understand if my situation has changed or if it's just different protocols/machines/doctors. I'm thrilled to have a better snapshot of my progress, so we can truly understand what is working and what's not and adjust as necessary.

We've been following the strict Vegan diet (no animal products, no gluten, no sugars, no alcohol), and it's going well. I'm not as panicked about every single thing I put in my mouth (I indulged in tortilla chips with my guacamole while out with my mom and sister, even though I'm quite sure they were deep fried in 'bad' oil), but I'm still careful to stay on course the majority of the time.

I have a wonderful new habit of exercising, then dry skin brushing, then meditating in the Infrared sauna for about 30 minutes every day! It feels like I'm doing something proactive, and it's super cleansing and centering.

I'm down to my last 2 Mistletoe shots and a few pills of

Artemisinin. I'm also taking Vitamin D and a Vegan Omega-3 daily, along with a few other gut healing drops.

I switched to a new provider of IV drips because he offered everything that I was given in Germany! We were excited to find him, and jumped in with both feet - starting with an aggressive 75 grams of vitamin C (I'd never done more than 50 grams) with an array of B vitamins and other minerals, Ozone Therapy (he'd remove my blood and inject it with Ozone then drip it back into my veins), and Artemisinin via IV.

Unfortunately, I had some pretty severe and disturbing reactions each time I got his infusions (once a week for 3 weeks). West has to drive me and sit with me for hours because it was so bad the first time, and it was incredibly difficult (and dangerous) for me to drive home - I couldn't lift my arms or hold my head up, I had a crushing headache, and I passed out hard for an hour each time. We tried removing the Magnesium and tried eating more carbs during treatment, but nothing helped. I'm going to take this as a sign from my body that this is not the right doctor for me!! We have an appointment this week at a new clinic, and I hope it goes better. It's almost twice the cost, but I honestly don't ever want to feel that way again... it felt like my heart was going to stop beating!

So that's the latest. We'll update here again after we get the test results on the 12th. Keep those healing vibes coming! XOXO"

LIFE IS COMPLICATED

"BALANCE is our ability to be flexible in the face of constant change" ~ **Louise L. Hay**

We had learned the hard way that stress was a strong contributor to the cancer. I had been doing everything I could to keep my stress to a minimum, and West was doing his best to be "Mr. Mom", but even Superman has his limits.

His sister was scheduled to have a fairly straightforward outpatient surgery on October 30. West asked me if he could take her to the hospital, and wait while she recovered - he said she had good friends nearby who could drive her, but he felt like he should be there. Of course, I said yes – she is family and she needed him. I would be fine alone for the day.

His sister lives about 45 minutes from us and lives alone, so it was important that he was there for her. She also lives on the 3rd floor of a walk-up, so she'd need his assistance getting back up to her apartment once the surgery was done.

Well, things didn't go as planned, and there were complications. They insisted that she stay at the hospital overnight for observation, and of course, West stayed with her until visiting hours were over, to keep her company and get her whatever she needed. He even went to her condo to take care of her two cats (yes, he'd do anything for family – even take care of a CAT!) If you know West, you know what a big deal that is).

When he called to tell me that he wouldn't be coming home that afternoon, it threw me a bit. Nonetheless, I needed to put on my 'big girl panties' and be responsible for the kids, which meant homework, dinner, sibling fights, bedtime, etc. I thought, "Ok, I can do this. It's only a couple of hours." I mean, my husband had traveled for work for the first 8 years of our kids' lives, and I had handled most everything on the home front, so I'd been in the trenches and survived. And this was only one evening.

But I'll be honest – I was nervous about taking the reins again, even if it was just for one day... My life was now ultra-focused on healing this unpredictable cancer, and I didn't know how to make room for anything else.

As most moms would do, I jumped in with both feet. I took all of my scheduled healing activities off of my calendar and headed to the store to buy some groceries for dinner. I checked homework and drove the kids to their horseback riding lesson and ninja class. We ate dinner and then headed off to bed. I was exhausted from all of the running around that I was no longer used to doing, but I made it through.

West came home late that first night, long after the kids had gone to bed. We sat up and talked about how his sister was doing, and what the next day might look like.

His sister was expecting to be released from the hospital the next morning once her stats had stabilized, and she wanted West to pick her up and get her settled at home. However, I also had my first appointment scheduled at a new IV clinic at the same time that morning... I would be receiving Ozone Therapy and high-dose vitamin C. West had planned to go with me in case I had any reactions and wasn't able to drive myself home safely, like my experiences with the last 3 infusions at the previous clinic.

I could tell that he was torn. He wanted to be there to support me, but he also felt like he needed to be there for his sister. I told him that he should do what he needed to do – I would be fine.

It's hard to admit, but I was hoping he'd *choose* to be with me. We'd been through a particularly rocky patch since the stressful event in August, and it was feeling unusually significant that he "pick me"– I needed to know that he would put me first, put our marriage first, even when it's hard. Perhaps it's not fair, but that's how I was feeling.

HALLOWEEN

"My to-do list for today:
Count my blessings; Practice kindness;
Let go of what I can't control: Listen to my heart; Be
productive yet calm; Just breathe."
~ Author Unknown

My infusion appointment was scheduled for 9:30 am at Thrive in Schaumburg, about a 20-minute drive from our house. We were still waiting to hear from West's sister about her discharge papers, and what time she'd be released from the hospital.

West felt that he needed to take care of his sister and get her settled. This had been an unnerving experience for her, and his presence would be reassuring. I wanted to support him in this, but I also desperately didn't want to be alone – I had my own unnerving experience at the previous IV clinic, and was fearful that I could have an equally disturbing experience at this new clinic. It was a conundrum, to be sure.

If you've ever been in the hospital, you know that getting

discharged rarely happens quickly. It was 9 am and there was no word from his sister about her timing. So I suggested to West that he drive me to my appointment, and if he got the call and needed to leave, then I would take an Uber home once my infusion was finished.

I loved the doctor and nurses at the new clinic, and it was a lovely space – clean and welcoming. was relieved that I felt pretty good after the infusions - a little tired, but no major reactions like I was having the previous 3 weeks with Dr. J.

West was able to stay with me for the entire infusion, and we drove home together. He dropped me off and then headed to the hospital in hopes that his sister would be released soon, and he'd be able to get back home to take the kids trick-or-treating after school. We were hoping to keep things as close to normal for them, especially on a holiday like this that is all about the kids.

Since I was feeling ok, I hopped in my car and headed to my lymphatic drainage appointment down the road. The kids got home from school shortly after I returned and were anxious to get their costumes on and head out with their pumpkins to gather goodies. However, there was still no word on when West might return.

I decided to pile the kids in the car and head to a friend's street nearby where there are sidewalks, and the houses are closer together. The kids could spend some time with their friends, and hopefully West would be home by the time we returned around dinner. He ended up staying with his sister through the evening and got home after the kids and I were all in bed. It was a very long day for both of us.

When I got the diagnosis in June, West was between jobs. He immediately stepped up and took over all of the shopping, meal planning, cooking, laundry, homework duties, driving the kids to various activities – he even started planning the play dates. I was able to focus all of my energy on healing, and dealing with the fear of the unknown. But without notice, the childcare and household duties unexpectedly fell back on my shoulders, and much to my surprise, it took its toll on me.

I could feel the stress building up over those two days, and though I rolled with the punches, I wasn't used to managing these kinds of stresses anymore. I was more fragile than I wanted to admit.

THE WATER FAST

"One reason people resist change is because they focus on what they have to give up, instead of what they have to gain." ~ Rick Godwin

Anxiety set in about the upcoming ultrasound, and I became fearful that the stress of the last few days might have fueled the tumor growth even more. I was feeling more and more desperate with each passing day...

Was there possibly more I could be doing that I hadn't yet added to my daily protocol?

I'd been reading a lot about water fasts and the power they have to help the body heal itself. You drink nothing but water for the duration of the fast, which typically lasts from 3 – 40 days. Water fasts have been around for centuries - in fact many religious traditions incorporate some form of fasting. I was intrigued...

There were many people in my cancer support groups who had used water fasting before, during, and after they received chemotherapy, so I'd been a part of many discussions surrounding the benefits of fasting. Researchers believe that fasting may make cancer cells more responsive to chemo while protecting the healthy cells, and it reduced the severity of the side effects from the harsh treatments. Amazing that such a simple thing as limiting your intake to water could have such powerful effects!

Fasting is essentially a form of detoxification, an opportunity to reset and reboot the body. Research shows that water fasting can reduce oxidative stress and boost the immune system – both vital when healing cancer naturally. It aids the body in clearing out damaged cells and replacing them with healthy new cells. Bingo!

I discussed these points with West to get his thoughts. He hesitated for a moment because I had already lost so much weight, but in the end he agreed that I should try it, and said he'd do it with me.

According to Steiner Health, "Probably the most important reason (to fast) is that the body uses quite a bit of energy to digest food, and when fasting this energy becomes available for other uses. In the fasting state, the body will scour for dead cells, damaged tissues, fatty deposits, tumors, abscesses, all of which are burned for fuel or expelled as waste. The elimination of these obstructions restores the immune system functionality and metabolic process to an optimum state."

WHEN THE BODY SPEAKS...

NOVEMBER 4, 2018

"If the plan doesn't work, change the plan, but never the goal." ~ Author Unknown

The first day of the water fast wasn't fun, but it was bearable. We drank A LOT of water, as well as plain herbal tea. I had a headache that developed as the day went on, but that was to be expected at the beginning of a fast.

In some ways, it made life simpler – there were no decisions to be made about what to eat, and no attention to the clock for guidance on when to eat. Yes, we still had the kids to think about, but they have their go-to favorites, and honestly, they were pretty happy they didn't have to 'try a bite' of the Vegan Shepherd's Pie or kale salad mom and dad typically ate.

Day 2 was a little more challenging. You start to get really hungry, and the intense cravings kick in. You long to chew something and experience the flavors of food. But we were doing this in the name of health, so we suffered...umm...I mean, *ventured* on!

Energy is quite low when starting a fast, so we had planned to take it easy for a few days. And good thing we did – I already had been having challenges with low energy reserves over the past few months, but now without any calories, I was beginning to feel depleted. I noticed that my arms got really tired in the shower while washing my hair – holding them above my head was exhausting.

Well that can't be a good sign.... Maybe I had lost too much weight to be doing something as dramatic as a water fast?

West seems to have an easier time with these sort of things. When he sets his mind to something, there's no stopping him. He's very black and white – he likes rules and will stick to them consistently without wavering.

I'd like to think I'm the same way – when I set a goal, I will do most anything I need to do to accomplish that goal. The difference is that I often course-correct – if something doesn't feel right along the way, I'll adjust my sails and switch directions.

I was starting to feel like this water fast might be too much for me...

On the third day of the water fast (the morning of Nov 6), I woke up feeling quite ill. I was weak and had a terrible headache. I tried to get out of bed, but I didn't have the strength to stand without a lot of effort. I had trouble walking to the bathroom.

My body was telling me that this was not the right thing for me at this point. I stopped the water fast and immediately drank a giant glass of fresh green juice – my body was craving nutrients, so that's what I gave it. I continued drinking fresh juices until my ultrasound and blood draw the following day.

SCANXIETY SETS IN

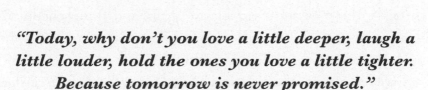

"Today, why don't you love a little deeper, laugh a little louder, hold the ones you love a little tighter. Because tomorrow is never promised."
~ Author Unknown

November 7, 2018 - the day of the follow up ultrasound and blood draw.

These tests always create something we Cancer Thrivers call "Scanxiety" – you can't help but feel anxious as the test day draws near. Will the tumor be smaller? Or will it show that the disease has progressed? Will they find something you didn't even know was there??

The last time I was facing these fears head on was in September, when the ultrasound showed that the tumor had grown to 3.2 cm, compared to 2.4 cm at my last scan in Germany on July 27. I was desperately hoping my efforts had been successful in turning things around, and we would see a smaller tumor.

Unfortunately, the results were not what we were hoping for – in fact, they were downright depressing. The tumor had continued to grow and was now 3.9 cm – bigger than it had ever been.

The news hit me really hard. It didn't seem to matter that I was 100% committed to a clean anti-cancer diet, or that I got IV infusions every week at $500 a crack, or that I was giving myself injections of Mistletoe Extract twice a week, or that I was getting daily exercise, using my sauna and BioMat, and doing meditation, or that I'd eliminated all the stress that I could from my life... the cancer was *growing*. And I was terrified.

It felt imperative that I get back into serious treatments at Marinus right away. Thankfully, we had already planned our trip after the previous disappointing scan, and were scheduled to leave in a week - PHEW! Knowing I'd be back in treatments made the bad news a little less crushing.

We met with the oncologist on November 12 and she confirmed the numbers from the ultrasound. It wasn't good news, but she wasn't giving up on me.

The blood test results actually showed that the CA-15-3 levels had come down a bit, and all other levels were in a good range. We tried to focus on the small victories.

We agreed to reassess once we returned from Germany in mid-December and see if we needed to adjust any elements of our protocol. Hopefully 3 weeks of intense daily treatments at the clinic would turn this ship around and get us back on track.

THE GREECE TEST

"New knowledge is the most valuable commodity on earth. The more truth we have to work with, the richer we become." ~ **Kurt Vonegut**

I had been hearing about another blood test that can offer insights into effective treatment options. It's called the RGCC test and is sometimes called the Greece Test, mainly because the only lab doing it is located in Greece. Several friends from Marinus had it done and found it helpful.

The Greece Test measures Circulating Tumor Cells (CTCs), which are cells that have detached from the primary tumor and flow into the blood or lymphatic circulation. These are the troublemakers that create secondary tumors or metastases in distant organs. CTCs, as well as CSCs (Cancer Stem Cells), are also responsible for cancer recurrence.

The test also provides information about the efficacy of natural biological substances or extracts on the cancer cells derived from a specific patient – it's customized medicine.

Having that information could turn out to be very valuable when considering what to add to my protocol, or what to remove.

I had been adding in so many elements, and it was getting overwhelming, time-consuming, and expensive. I felt like I was grasping at straws at times. There are no clear answers when it comes to cancer, and it's nearly impossible to know for certain what is having an effect and what isn't. If this simple blood test could tell us that, for instance, high-dose vitamin C and Ozone Therapy had absolutely no effect on my type of cancer, then we could remove those treatments – that change alone would save us nearly two thousand dollars a month.

I did ask the doctor where I get my IV infusions if he had heard of the Greece Test, and he said he could order it for me. He would draw my blood and overnight it to the lab in Greece. However, he charged $4,500... holy cow. I had heard that Dr. Weber could order the same test for half the cost. I would wait and discuss this test with Dr. W. once I arrived in Germany.

EUROPE—HERE WE COME

NOVEMBER 16, 2018

"Note to self: RELAX. You are enough. You do enough. Breathe extra deep, let go and just live right now in the moment." ~ **Author Unknown**

We were headed to Europe!

West and I decided to take the kids along with us for this second trip to Marinus. I not only wanted the company (it was hard not seeing my kids for 3 weeks during my last trip, and if I'm honest, a little scary to make this journey all alone), I also wanted to expose them to other cultures.

I suggested that we fly straight into Amsterdam and spend a day or two there, so I could show the kids where I had spent 5 years of my life in the 90's.

We flew out of Chicago on Friday night, trying desperately to sleep on the plane (no easy task), and arrived in Amsterdam around 9 am local time. We grabbed a taxi to the hotel to drop off our bags and then headed out on foot to explore.

We found an inexpensive hotel near Dam Square, only

minutes from the main train station. I had booked us on a special "pirate themed" canal cruise geared towards kids, so we decided to meander through the streets headed toward Leidse-plein, where we would board the canal boat.

It was chilly in Amsterdam in November, but luckily the sun was shining, and it felt really good to be walking after sitting on a plane for over 10 hours. And there were lots of things to see! It brought back memories of my time spent on those streets oh so many years ago.

We made it to the boat with time to spare, so we stopped by a small kiosk along the canal to purchase some fresh fruit and stroopwafels (waffle cookies held together with honey or syrup), my kids' favorite traditional Dutch treat. ☺ Boy, did that make them happy!

We all enjoyed the tour throughout the many canals of this amazing city, and the kids were fascinated with the architecture. When we returned, West lead us to a Vegan restaurant nearby to grab some lunch (good thing those kids had already eaten!)

Later that afternoon, we took a train up to Hoorn, a cute little town about 45 minutes north of Amsterdam where I lived for the last 2 years of my stay in Holland. We had dinner with some old friends who also had children, and we were delighted to see how well they all got along! It was fun watching them teach each other English and Dutch. ☺

With our bellies full and our hearts content, we headed back to our little hotel for a good night's sleep.

HOLLAND, MY OLD HOME

NOVEMBER 18, 2018

"Be grateful for what you have, and where you are in your journey.
Gratitude is key to manifesting abundance."
~ Abraham Hicks

Day 2: Our adventures in Holland continue!

It's amazing how you can find healthy options anywhere if you just look! We found a fresh juice place only steps from our hotel, so that's where we decided to go for a good breakfast to start our 2nd day. They also offered healthy versions of waffles and typical kid-pleasing fare with lots of fresh fruit, so everyone was happy.

We then walked to the train station and hopped on a train to Zaanse Schans near Haarlem – an adorable town reminiscent of the 18th and 19th centuries in Holland, full of wooden houses, mills, barns, and workshops. This magical place was always on the agenda when friends would visit me from the States, so of course, I wanted my kids to experience it!

We spent the entire day there, walking through working windmills, witnessing a tree trunk become wooden clogs before our eyes, learning how cheese is made and tasting many samples (Langdon was in heaven!), and touring the village.

We stopped into the local eatery for pannenkoeken, a type of Dutch pancake that is thin and wide and typically stuffed with yummy things. You can choose savory fillings like ham and cheese or sweet fillings like apples and cinnamon (yep, those are the two versions my kids got). West and I had vegetable soup and tea.

When it was time to head back to Amsterdam, we boarded the train and accidentally sat in the first class section near the conductor. The conductor was a very kind man who came out to chat with the kids. He said we could stay since there weren't many people on the train, and then invited the kids into his cab to help him announce over the intercom that we had arrived in Amsterdam! Imagine the surprise when the passengers heard a young girl's voice say it in English. Addison had a huge grin on her face for an hour!

West had done quite a bit of research on Vegan restaurants in Amsterdam and found a little place near our hotel, so we walked over to grab some dinner. It was an interesting hole in the wall with only 5 tables, one of which was on the floor with pillows – which is, of course, where we sat. The food was decent, though it took forever. We were certain the man taking our order was also the cook!

We wandered the streets for a while and eventually stopped at an ice cream shop to get a treat for the kids before heading back to the hotel to pack and get to sleep. We would be heading to Munich on an early flight the next morning.

BRANNENBURG

NOVEMBER 19, 2018

"Worrying won't stop the bad stuff from happening.
It just stops you from enjoying the good."
~ Winnie the Pooh

We were off to Brannenburg for my 2nd round of treatments!

We arrived at the Munich airport, and the car sent from Marinus took us to the little apartment we had rented about a 30-minute walk from the clinic. It had 2 bedrooms, a bathroom/shower combo, a small kitchen with a table and chairs, and a small living area – perfect for a family of four.

Once we got settled, the whole family walked over to the clinic so I could get started with treatments.

It felt good to be back at the clinic, in a place that was healing and peaceful. After all of the ups and downs over the previous 5 months, I needed to refocus and hopefully shrink this darn tumor.

One of the first things they do is draw blood to check levels, and then you visit Dr. Helena to get an ultrasound. My last ultrasound was less than 2 weeks prior and showed that the tumor had grown to 3.9 cm. We were anxious to see what today's scan would show.

On the bright side, Dr. Helena scanned my lymph nodes, liver, pancreas, gallbladder, and other various organs in my midsection, and everything looked clear.

On the not-so-bright side, she measured the tumor and it was now 4.1 cm... Boy, was I glad I was at a cancer clinic - we needed to put the brakes on this sucker and fast!!

I met with Dr. Weber to discuss the blood test results and create a plan for my 3 weeks of treatments. There were a few issues that needed to be addressed:

My hemoglobin was low, and after comparing it to labs from previous months, we discovered that it had been continually dropping since my treatments in July. Dr Weber had learned that this was potentially caused by the Artemisinin, and suggested we stop it immediately. My levels returned to a healthy range after the first week. Artemisinin would no longer be a part of my protocol.

We also discovered that my liver enzymes were slightly elevated again. I had experimented with adding the mushroom supplements back in, but now I know they are causing problems. The mushrooms must go, for good! My liver is clearly sensitive and gets overwhelmed when it has to process too many pills (even if they are natural and not pharmaceuticals). I will aim at getting most of my needs covered with food or IV's. A benefit of IV therapy is that it goes directly into your bloodstream and doesn't need to be processed by the organs.

On a positive note, the CA-15-3 came down to 26 from the high of 33 in September – at least something was headed in the right direction.

A DARK & COLD WALK HOME

♥

"Seek healing, a refilling of energy and spirit, as soon as you see that you need it.
You don't have to push yourself to give, do, or perform when what your body, mind, soul and emotions need is to heal."
~ Melody Beattie

I ended up staying quite late on that first day at the clinic to fit in all of my treatments. I didn't get out of Hyperthermia until 8 pm, long after the sun had gone down.

Unfortunately, there are no street lights in this quaint little dairy village, and the walk back to the apartment was dark, cold and a little scary, to be honest. I called West on my cell phone and asked him to meet me halfway. I was worn out from the flight as well as from the treatments, and couldn't wait to get back to our "home away from home" and get some rest...

Thankfully, the staff at the clinic was able to schedule all remaining treatments to be completed by 4 pm so I could get back to my family and enjoy some 'together' time, which also meant that I could get back before sundown.

My post to the private FB group on November 21, 2018:

"It's much colder here in Brannenburg than it was in July, obviously, so no more yoga in the garden for me! The colorful flowers are gone, and my peaceful mountain is mostly covered by low fog...

Monday was a long day of traveling, meeting with Dr Weber, starting treatments, and settling into our/my home for the next 3 weeks.

Medical updates:

I won't bore you all with the list of treatments I'm getting as they are mostly the same as my last visit. If you want to be reminded, scroll down to one of our previous posts from July - West did a great job at describing what was done and why.

We had our first ultrasound with Helena. The good news is that there were still no signs of any spread to other organs or lymph nodes. I'm clinging to any good news I can get!

The tumor measured 4.1 cm (the largest so far), which is troubling, but we're hopeful that these treatments will have an impact, and the final scan will show shrinkage by the end of my trip. The measurement is similar to what we got in Hinsdale two weeks ago (3.9 cm), so that tells us that the machines and findings are similar.

Sadly this means that the tumor was indeed shrinking in June and July (the last ultrasound in Germany showed 2.4 cm), but has been growing rapidly since August... darn...

I did have some incredibly stressful life events in August and September, so I thought that might have been a slight detour on our path, but we can't seem to turn this ship around...

Dr L., my Integrative Oncologist in Hinsdale, said that the cancer gets "smart" over time and figures out ways to thrive, even with all of our efforts and lifestyle changes (she said this also happens with chemo - it will work for a time, but then things will change - it's an insidious disease). We are trying some new approaches and hope to see improvement over the next 2 months.

We've run into a few of our friends (fellow patients) from our last visit, and made a few more. Lots of folks from New Zealand (a 23-hour journey here!!) and from America (Tennessee, Wisconsin, Minnesota, Texas, to name a few).

Overall, not much worse than what was expected. I'll get another blood test next week, and we'll adjust as necessary.

Please keep us in your thoughts and continue to send those healing vibes! And thanks for following along on my healing journey! Love to you all."

ADVENTURES BEFORE THE FAMILY DEPARTS

"When 'I' is replaced with 'We', even illness becomes wellness." ~ **Malcolm X**

Snow, rain, cold... the walks to and from the apartment were long and unpleasant, and a little draining after a full day of treatments.

I rented a bike from the clinic in hopes of making it easier. The ride home was mostly downhill and, on a bike, only took 15 minutes. However, the ride to the clinic in the morning was conversely uphill and it became a bit tough in the rain and snow... Each day, I felt more exhausted than the day before.

On the other hand, my family was here in Germany with me and they were patiently filling their days while I was at the clinic. I needed to summon the energy to explore Bavaria with them!

Unfortunately, our beautiful mountain was "closed" the entire time we were there - it was between seasons, and they were preparing for the skiers who would soon be arriving upon this glorious mountain. No cog train ride for the kids...

We rented some bikes for the kids and rode into Brannen-burg to do some shopping one afternoon. On another day, we took the train to Rosenheim and had dinner at the Indian restaurant that West and I had found on our previous trip. We also ventured into Austria! It was only a 10-minute train ride to another country, and the station was only a few minutes from our apartment.

Kufstein is a cute little city complete with a fortress on a hill. We heard that there was a torture chamber inside, so of course we had to check it out. Honestly, it was pretty disturbing...it was hard to believe that people were tortured in despicable ways simply for not subscribing to the norm. Boy, would I have been in trouble!

We enjoyed a traditional Bavarian feast for dinner (well, the kids had Schnitzel and fries, and we had a "gemuzeteller", otherwise known as a vegetable plate) before returning to Brannenburg to pack up for their departure the next day.

I was really going to miss having the kids around and hearing their giggles. And I was absolutely going to miss West and everything he had been doing to make sure we were all taken care of...

THANKSGIVING

NOVEMBER 22, 2018

"In the blink of an eye, everything can change.
So forgive often and love with all your heart.
You never know when you may not have the chance
again." ~ Author Unknown

My post to the private FB group:

"Goodness...my heart hurts...

I just met a lovely couple from Ireland. They were so friendly, and we were chatting in the sitting area in the clinic. Eventually, I asked which one of them was the patient here. That's when they told me that their daughter was the patient, but she died last night...

That hit me so hard. I hugged the mother and couldn't stop the tears from coming. It's just not right when a child dies before the parent. I can't even imagine losing my daughter...

Later that day, I met the deceased patient's older sister who was making funeral plans. The whole family was meeting at Marinus because this place had meant so very much to her sister. She shared a bit of the story with me: her sister found a lump in her breast 5 years ago. She had been coming to Marinus for treatments for 3 years and was doing really well. She had chosen to treat her cancer holistically – no chemo, radiation or surgery.

Then 2 months ago, things took a terrible turn, and the cancer metastasized to her organs. They tried to do emergency surgery, but it was too late...

She was young and had 4 children who have now lost their mother – this crushes my heart... So many people see progress here and heal, but the sad truth is that not everyone survives... this disease is invasive and consumes you. If you are lucky, you overcome. And it changes your life completely, forever.

I read a passage recently that said, "*Life* is a terminal condition. None of us survive it. It is just a matter of how and when we will die." Such a true statement, but so often we are too busy to realize that we all have a limited amount of time on this earth. We must make the most of every moment.

This was a true reminder to be grateful for each and every day that we are given. None of us are promised tomorrow. Without warning, your entire future can change. Be thankful, especially today, for everything good in your life. And above all, be thankful for those wonderful people in your life who love you just because of who you are - I know I am so very thankful every day for all of you."

THE COWGIRL FROM TEXAS

"Do the best you can until you know better.
Then, when you know better, do better."
~ Maya Angelou

While getting therapy in the common space, I overheard someone talking about a friend (let's call her T), whom I met in July. We had kept in touch, and we discovered that our stays at Marinus were going to overlap by a week! I was excited to see T again.

I heard the Australian woman mention my friend's name, so I asked where T was since I hadn't seen her, and it had been a few days. She gave me the saddest look, and I knew something was wrong...

When I met T last July, I liked her instantly. T always had a smile on her face and a sunny outlook, even though she was terrified of this disease.

She had discovered a small lump in her right breast 2 years

earlier and had come to Marinus to heal naturally. The treatments successfully eliminated any sign of cancer from her body!

T told us that she then returned to Texas and went back to her old life filled with stress and fast food. After 2 years of being on the road and not taking care of herself, the lump returned with a vengeance, and now she was back at Marinus for treatments again.

When I met T in July, the lump had grown to several centimeters in diameter. Unfortunately, the cancer had also metastasized and was now in her bones and liver. She was concerned, but was seeing progress with the treatments here.

She returned home with a different perspective of healthy living and vowed to do what she could to keep this under control.

West and I took her story to heart – once you receive a cancer diagnosis, even if there are no more signs of disease, your everyday choices MATTER. This truth would ring in my head each and every day going forward.

LOSING A FRIEND

"Everyone you meet is fighting a battle you know nothing about. Be kind. Always." ~ **Brad Meltzer**

After only 4 months at home, T came back to Marinus in November to tackle some disturbing symptoms – the tumor seemed to be growing out of her chest. It was red and hot to the touch, and she was worried.

My new Australian friend had arrived around the same time as T, and they were staying at the same bed and breakfast.

As she and I sat in the common area, she shared the events of the past few days. She told me that T had not been doing well after she arrived, and eventually Dr. W. insisted that she stay in the clinic and not make the walk from the bed and breakfast – it was too much on her struggling body.

My friend told me how she and T would dine together at the clinic. At times, she was her typical happy self, but at other times, she would slip away suddenly - she'd stop mid-sentence, and her eyes would glaze over. It seemed that the tumor had grown out of control and became infected, and the infection had traveled to her brain...

Dr. W. could see that she now needed help beyond the scope of the clinic. He sent her to a nearby hospital where they could hopefully get the infection under control. Her mom flew to Germany to be by her side, but they eventually decided it would be best to get medical transport to fly her home to Texas so she could be with her husband and young boys.

On Sunday, November 25, West and the kids left Germany and flew back home to Chicago, leaving me alone in the apartment we had rented. After I gave them all kisses and watched their car drive away, I biked to the clinic for my morning treatments.

On my way to the treatment room, I ran into my Australian friend. She stopped me with a gentle touch on my arm, and I knew instantly... She then softly shared that T had landed in Texas and died 4 hours later, before her boys could get to her side.

I went numb.

I could hardly believe she was really gone... she seemed so positive and full of life in July, only a few months prior. How did this all happen so quickly??

I finished my treatments early and returned to the empty apartment in Flintsbach. I sat there in the stark living room for the rest of the day, alone. I felt emotions spilling out from the depths of my soul – sadness over the loss of my friend, vulnerability because we walked similar paths, intense fear that her story may eventually be my own...

She was only 46 - a mother with young kids, just like me. Only 2 short years ago, she was living her life freely, having no idea that she only had a short amount of time left on this earth.

SWIRLING THOUGHTS

"You are not supposed to be happy all the time. Life hurts and it's hard. Not because you're doing it wrong, but because it hurts for everybody. Don't avoid the pain. You need it. It's meant for you. Be still with it, let it come, let it go, let it leave you with the fuel you'll burn to get your work done on this earth."
~ Glennon Doyle Melton

I had bouts of uncontrollable sobbing throughout the day and was spiraling out of control. It was hard being alone. But sitting in that room without anyone around to console me actually allowed me to feel everything completely, which is the only true way to heal. I was feeling the raw emotions without having to temper them for anybody.

It was cathartic and cleansing, and it gave me the quiet

space I needed to think about my own situation and the decisions before me.

I had been considering having a lumpectomy, but until this point, wasn't sure if it was the right move for me. Surgery is stressful and puts a huge load on the body and the immune system, something I was desperately trying to reduce. Surgery also comes with its own risks, like lymphedema, infections, or issues with anesthesia.

Hearing details of T's final days and knowing the choices she had made along the way, I contemplated the possibility of having the tumor in my right breast removed. It was becoming clear that I may not be able to eliminate it on my own, and perhaps T's story was meant to shine a light on the fact that cancer can switch directions and spread quickly. I knew this, of course, but losing a friend made it very real...

I couldn't help but wonder...had T crossed my path on this journey for a reason? Had she come into my life at this moment in time to teach me something?

THE LONGEST DAY OF MY LIFE

♥

"Not all storms come to disrupt your life. Some come to clear your path." ~ **Author Unknown**

I reached out to my brother, who happens to be a licensed psychologist, hoping he could help me work through the numerous terrifying thoughts zipping around my brain. We texted back and forth throughout the day, and I was so very grateful for his understanding and gentle approach.

In hopes of helping other Cancer Thrivers, and with his permission, I'm sharing the conversation I had with my brother below. His wise words were incredibly helpful in some of my darkest hours.

Me: "I'm hoping you can offer some guidance... I've been having emotional moments a lot here lately. Moments of deep sadness... it's challenging to stay positive. Especially when some of my friends/fellow patients here are dying. I'm so incredibly scared... I'm feeling so conflicted about what to do. These friends were just like me - committed to the natural path. But their paths took sudden detours and there was no turning back at that point..."

J (my brother): "My dear sweet sister, thank you for confiding with me. I would be most proud if I could find a way to be helpful. My thoughts:

I'm sorry about your friends and how sad that is for you, and I'm sorry that you are so scared that this may say something about your own possible fate; but neither of these are incorrect emotions. They are the ways you are supposed to feel. I am sad and scared for you, too.

The usual antidote for sadness is grieving and mourning. This might seem like the opposite of positive, but it's not. I think it's more akin to acceptance and embracing sorrow (always about some form of loss) than it is a form of pessimism (which is really about predicting the future as negative, not necessarily facing the present). We will sometimes not begin to grieve for ourselves or others until we have to, and sometimes not even then.

The antidote for fear is comfort and restoration of safety (the former I hope you have; the latter may not be readily available). Fear is a great motivator - it energizes us to move to safety (again, when that's available, and it doesn't stop us from trying when it's not). That leaves a big question: safety from what?

As much as you may have benefited from being positive and dedicated and doing everything you can to make yourself healthy again, I wonder if that has also left you vulnerable and unprepared for setbacks.

I take it that you're rethinking your choices regarding your cancer treatment. I support that. From what I can tell, you have kept your options open and have been responsible in informing yourself and seeking a wide range of professional input. I don't have an opinion about what is best for you, but you would certainly have my support if you decided to change course.

Sorry this is so long winded, and probably way more intellectualized than you want or need. I'm guessing I haven't said anything you didn't already know. Much love, let's keep talking."

Me: "No it was perfect. Just the perspective I needed."

Me: "I am considering many things, and have been doing much research, as I always have, but expanding the options since the tumor started growing again a few months ago.

The recent loss of friends is indeed adding a fear element to my decisions - would they still be here if they had made a different choice? If they hadn't waited so long? Is it somehow a sign that I need to remove the tumor while I have a chance? Before it gets so large it's impossible or before it spreads and complicates things?

At times, surgery feels like the right thing to do - at other times, it feels like a decision made out of fear. It's something that can't be un-done, so I need to be sure.

The doctor here is worried that my type of cancer isn't responding well, and is recommending a drug that supposedly doesn't have major side effects, but I know in my soul how pharmaceuticals can mess up your immune system. Again, that would be a decision made from fear... at least at this point. I've found a lot of people who have taken both routes and am gathering information-both useful and scary.

The unknown is what is terrifying me..."

J: "What is known at this point? (not rhetorical, actual question)"

Me: "The tumor was shrinking rapidly in the first months. Then in September, tests showed it had reversed and was growing rapidly and still continues to grow...

My cancer markers were normal in July. In September, they had more than doubled into troublesome territory. They have lowered a bit over the last month, but the tumor is at its largest measured size.

My energy is low on most days, and I've lost 31 pounds since the diagnosis. Luckily it has stabilized now, but I've lost a lot of muscle mass.

My days are filled with healing treatments and there is very little time left for fun or actual living... just trying to manage these modalities and this incredibly restrictive diet is exhausting."

J: "Could surgery be the right thing and still be based on fear?

I worry about your weakness and weight loss; I worry that there is a window that could close. But... I respect everything you're doing, and I am not a fan of traditional Western medicine in so many regards and will always choose to avoid surgery where I can. Then again, I've never faced what you're facing, and you're sounding like this is all covered territory for you. I will say, I'm less worried now about the clarity of your thinking. So, that's a good thing!"

Me: "Yes, I do believe surgery could be the right decision, even if it's based on fear. After all, there's a lot of fear connected to cancer and the very real possibility of dying!

I also worry about my weakness... it's very frustrating when I'm not able to get through a yoga class that used to be so vital to my health.

And I too am very concerned that there is a window that might close... the woman who died a few days ago (young mother of 4 children) had been successful on the natural path for 3 years, then 2 months ago, it took a nasty turn. They did an emergency surgery a few weeks later, and she wasn't able to recover...

The friend who died today was at the Klinik getting treatment, just last week. It got so bad she had to be admitted to the hospital here in Germany (she was also a mother of 2 boys the same ages as my kids), and she was too weak to have surgery.

Thank you so much for your support and your wise insights. It has been incredibly helpful to talk it out with someone who knows me, and who knows how to listen without judgment."

J: "N and I will be thinking about you; we are pulling for you and want for you to get strong again. Please share your thoughts (and fears), anytime. I want to know your decision making process, if you'd care to keep me posted. You are most loved."

30 YEARS OF FRIENDSHIP

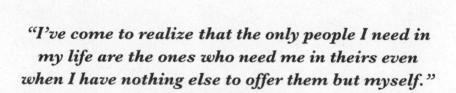

**"I've come to realize that the only people I need in my life are the ones who need me in theirs even when I have nothing else to offer them but myself."
~ Author Unknown**

My dear friend of 30 years, Jen, touched me beyond measure. When she heard that I was headed back to Marinus for another round of treatments, and learned that West was only staying with me for the first week this time, she selflessly made arrangements to come to Germany to be by my side for a few days so I wouldn't be alone. She left her own family and a full-time job to make the trip.

It was such a grand gesture of love and friendship, and it was so incredibly appreciated.

Even as I write this, months after the fact, it still brings tears to my eyes. I was so deeply humbled that someone would do that for me... leave life behind and cross the ocean to sit beside a friend. She took such good care of me, shopping and cooking, and keeping my spirits up. It was exactly what I needed after all that had happened recently.

The power of friendship is truly magical, and I am so very grateful for the people in my life who didn't hesitate for a second to be there when I needed them.

FITTING IN SOME ADVENTURE

"Things are never quite as scary when you've got a best friend." ~ **Bill Watterson**

What a fun-filled afternoon and evening in Salzburg!

I had treatments all morning, so after a delicious salmon lunch that Jen cooked, we hopped on a train for Austria and arrived an hour and half later. We hopped on a tour bus and took in the sites! We hopped off at an amazing Christmas market where we learned about Krampus (if you don't know about this unusual tradition, check it out!), and then hopped off again in Old Town to grab some dinner before heading back to Flintsbach. We packed in as much as a human can in a handful of hours!

We also made a trip to Kufstein, did a tour of the Riedel Factory where we witnessed jaw-dropping glass blowing techniques, and enjoyed a final dinner together near the fortress.

In addition to everything Jen did to support me, she also created an amazing opportunity for herself while I was in active treatments - she found a dance studio in Brannenburg and arranged to teach a Be Moved class! So proud of my amazing friend!! She connects with people everywhere she goes, and doesn't hesitate to spread her love of dance whenever possible! Nothing stands in her way of sharing her passion - not even a language barrier.

It's clear to me why we've been close for so many years. She's an all-around fabulous person, and I am so blessed to have her in my life!

THE ONLY CONSTANT IS CHANGE

"I love when people that have been through hell walk out of the flames carrying buckets of water for those still consumed by the fire."
~ **Stephanie Sparkles**

I am a member of several cancer support groups, one of which is Square 1, started by Chris Wark. This group focuses on diet and lifestyle changes, as well as many alternative holistic treatments for cancers of all kinds.

It is there that I connected with a new friend, B, who had also been diagnosed with triple negative breast cancer, and was a mother of young children. It's hard to find other Cancer Thrivers who have conquered triple negative, as it's often more aggressive and difficult to treat. We shared our stories and were inspiring to each other.

B was in remission and told me how she had seen clear changes in her numbers (cancer markers) with a strict Keto for Cancer diet. When she was committed to it, her numbers were in the normal range; when she'd "cheat" or get relaxed and eat too much of the foods that turn to sugar quickly, her numbers skyrocketed. She'd then recommit 100%, and her numbers would return to normal. She was, in essence, her very own science experiment, and could clearly see the difference her choices were making.

This sounded intriguing to me, especially now that the tumor was growing out of control. The lifestyle changes and the strict vegan diet that had been successfully reducing the tumor at the beginning were no longer having an effect. Perhaps this was the change that would help turn things around.

I spoke with Dr. Weber about this possible shift in my eating approach and he was enthusiastically supportive of it. I had been doing quite a bit of reading on the benefits of a Keto diet, especially for diseases such as cancer, and I was now convinced that it was worth a try.

On December 1, 2018, I switched to a Keto for Cancer approach.

The Ketogenic Diet is NOT a heavy meat diet, contrary to what many people think. The focus is on healthy fats like coconut oil and olive oil, nuts and nut butters, and avocado. Proteins are limited to only 20% of your total intake, which equates to 2 eggs and a piece of fish. Carbs are limited to 10%, and should come mainly from vegetables.

It also isn't an invitation to fill up on 'Keto-approved' foods that aren't actually healthy - like bacon, sausage, deli meats and pork rinds. I was determined to focus on colorful veggies with healthy fats, and smaller portions of meats and cheeses.

I would also treat myself to 5 or 6 berries a day - most fruit is a no-no on Keto, but berries are lower on the Glycemic Index. My friend B had done the calculations, and learned that more than a handful of berries may push you over the limit and out of Ketosis.

www.thetruthaboutcancer.com/plant-based-keto-diet

www.thetruthaboutcancer.com/ketogenic-diet-weakens-cancer-cells/comment-page-1

Does sugar feed cancer growth?

www.natureworksbest.com/blog/2014/05/27/sugar-feeds-cancer-growth

THE UNIVERSE SENDS YOU WHAT YOU NEED

"Sometimes the smallest step in the right direction ends up being the biggest step of your life. Tip toe if you must, but take the step."
~ Author Unknown

B lived near Munich, so we planned to meet in person while I was at the clinic. We decided we would meet on a Sunday since my treatments were done earlier on weekends, and we'd have more time to visit. She took the train to Brannenburg, and Jen and I met her at the station.

The 3 of us walked from the station to a coffee house nearby, and chatted over tea. We clicked instantly! I adored her positive spirit and her commitment to living life to the fullest while still managing this disease to make sure it never took hold again.

We talked about the ups and downs of this crazy journey, and discussed the potential pitfalls of the Keto approach. B had generously brought along a gift for me – The "Keto for Cancer"

Cookbook - and it would prove to be a lifesaver as I navigated this new path.

I am so grateful for her kindness and her invaluable knowledge that she gleaned from walking the path before me. Her guidance was and still is indispensable.

While at the coffee house, B reached into her bag and pulled out some Keto test strips and a breathing apparatus – she wanted to see if I was perhaps already in Ketosis (when your body begins to burn fat instead of sugar and releases Ketones into the blood).

Amazingly, the tests showed that I was indeed in Ketosis already! That's when the magic happens!

It had only been 2 days since the switch, but I had already been sugar-free for months, so it wasn't a huge shift in that sense. I did experience mild headaches, but nothing like the "Keto flu" that you hear about. Thankfully, this had been a pretty easy transition for me.

And I must admit – I was enjoying the new food options available to me. Instead of rice and quinoa (neither of which are very satisfying to me), I was now eating butter and fish! It was surreal when my first Keto meal arrived at the table and a WHOLE FISH, head and all, was plopped down in front of me! Quite a shock for someone who was Vegan only moments before... True, I could no longer eat potatoes, most fruits, or carrots and beets, but now I could have some pasture-raised chicken alongside the piles of vegetables, or a little cheese on my salad. I was embracing this change whole-heartedly.

About a week into the diet shift, we did a follow up ultrasound at the clinic, and it showed that the tumor had stabilized. Could it be that the Keto diet was halting the tumor growth??

Again, we don't know what we don't know - so in many ways it's a guessing game. Each and every cancer is different, and every patient's body will react differently. Some things will work for one person and not for the next – even if they have the exact same diagnosis. In my mind, it made sense to try the least harmful approaches first to see what had an impact on my particular situation.

I was so grateful that a combination of the diet shift and the myriad of holistic treatments at the clinic seemed to be changing the course of my disease.

**Check out B's Instagram posts for Keto inspiration! @Beebee_challenged

INTERMITTENT FASTING

"Your body will heal itself, through gentle and peaceful cooperation with the inherent wisdom and intelligence within." ~ **Bryant McGill**

I've been practicing Intermittent Fasting (IF) for many years – eating only between the hours of 11 am and 6:30 pm on most days. This is a great way to maintain a healthy weight, but it turns out it's also powerful for healing cancer.

"Research on the benefits of IF is now widespread. A 2013 study conducted by Thomas Jefferson University discovered that IF slowed the growth of primary cancer tumors, and also decreased the number of new ones in breast cancer patients.[9]"

www.thetruthaboutcancer.com/keto-for-wome

What is fasting and how does it help heal the body?

www.chrisbeatcancer.com/the-fast-lane-to-health

" *"What we have to recognize ... is that if cancer is a mitochondrial metabolic disease and you get cancer because of mitochondrial failure in certain populations of cells and certain tissues, if you prevent your mitochondria from entering into this dysfunctional state ... [then] the probability of getting cancer is going to be significantly reduced.*

To what percent? I would say a minimum of 80 percent. Cancer is probably, as I said in my book, one of the most manageable diseases that we know of...

The problem is that many people don't want [to take the preventive steps to avoid cancer]. They're like, 'I have to therapeutically fast for a week? Oh, I'm not going to. Give me a break' ... An effective prevention is to eat less and move more. A lot of people don't want to do that... Once you realize what cancer is, that it's a metabolic disease, you can take charge of those kinds of things. In other words, getting cancer is not God's will. It's not bad luck."

~ Dr. Thomas Seyfried

ADJUSTING THE APPROACH

NOVEMBER 30TH, 2018

"You must find the place inside yourself where nothing is impossible." ~ **Deepak Chopra**

I sent the following update to my brother:

Me: "I have decided to shift my diet starting tomorrow - instead of Vegan (which had an impact for the first few months, but isn't working anymore), I'm going to try Keto. A friend with my same diagnosis had great results, and she's coming here on Sunday to help guide me.

I'm also feeling more confident that I'm going to have the tumor removed in December. I believe it will remove a great deal of stress and pain. It is a constant reminder of my vulnerability and creates a bit of an obsession, and it makes it difficult to sleep or do yoga and such because of the pain. I've spoken to other patients, and they had great relief once the main tumor was gone.

If I see some good progress, I may put off the meds the doc is recommending - I just hate to poison my body... but I'll purchase the pills and take them home with me, so I have the option.

I haven't shared these possible paths with anyone, so please keep them to yourself until I make my final decisions, and am ready to share with the entire group/family. Love you."

SOMETIMES A SHIFT IS NECESSARY

*"Each person's journey is different. If something -
anything - does not feel right to you, then you alone
get to decide whether you will honor it or not. The
choice of how to respond to your situation is yours -
and will always be yours."*
~ **Susan Barbara Apollon**

My post to the private group:

"As most of you know, West and I were 100% dedicated to a Vegan diet from the day of my diagnosis. It (along with the other therapies we were doing) was having a terrific impact for the first few months - cancer markers stayed in the normal range and the tumor shrunk significantly.

However, things took a downward turn over the past few months, and last week we decided it was time to make a shift and hopefully turn it back around. I've often heard that you've got to keep cancer on its toes and switch things up once in a while!

We've added bloodroot to our protocol (it's supposed to attack the cancer cells from the inside), we've removed Artemisinin since it was negatively affecting my hemoglobin levels, I've changed some supplements, and we've switched to a Keto for Cancer Diet.

This has been mentally challenging for both of us after being so committed to absolutely no animal products... but we're encouraged by what we're seeing.

Ten days into the diet change and switches of supplements, and I'm happy to say that I'm experiencing less pain in my tumor and surrounding areas. That makes it easier to find a comfortable position for sleeping - phew!

It also means I'm not reminded of the cancer constantly, which is a very good thing for my mental health.

I've also gained 5 pounds! I've never in my life been excited about GAINING weight... until now. I lost a lot of weight on the Vegan diet, especially at the beginning, and was down to 113 pounds at one point (not healthy for a girl that's 5'9). I was lethargic and had trouble doing daily activities at times, so it was frustrating. But I'm starting to feel more human and my energy is returning little by little.

Triple negative breast cancer is particularly tricky and especially aggressive, so we needed to try something. We are hopeful that this shift will continue to have an impact.

So grateful to be here at Marinus, but I can't wait to get home to my family..."

UPDATE TIME

"And once the storm is over, you won't remember how you made it through, how you managed to survive. You won't even be sure whether the storm is really over. But one thing is certain. When you come out of the storm, you won't be the same person who walked in. That's what the storm's all about." ~ **Haruki Murakami**

My post to the private group after my visit to Germany:

"I had my final meeting with Dr. Weber. All of my blood-work is stable (hemoglobin back to normal, cancer markers the same, liver bounces around in a pretty normal range).

Tumor is pretty much the same size...4.1 cm. I'm a little bummed, but trying to see the positive side - these treatments have stopped it from growing. It was on a bad path, so I'll take what I can get.

I have a follow up with my oncologist next week, so we'll see if there's better news then, after my body has calmed down from all of these treatments. The doc who does the ultrasound said that an hour of hyperthermia every day can make the tumor swell, and it's impossible to tell how much is active tumor and what is swollen tissue. Maybe it's a little smaller, but not likely.

Dr. Weber seemed to think the tumor/cancer is stable for now, but we're clearly not making strides in eliminating it.

He's always been very open-minded and straight forward, which we appreciate. I told him that I've been considering surgery at the end of December, and he thought that was the right next step for me. In fact, he's been encouraging it since July, but I needed to do some soul searching, and make sure it was the right thing for me at this time.

We did our best to eliminate the cancer using only natural methods, but almost 6 months in and it's larger than it was at the start.

I've done a lot of thinking and researching, and have scheduled a lumpectomy with Dr. Winchester for December 26, so I can enjoy the holidays with my family before recovering.

I am fully aware that removing the tumor doesn't mean that I'm healed. One important thing I've learned on this journey is that I will always be vulnerable to cancer, so it's imperative that I continue with my therapies and healthy living to address any cancer cells swimming elsewhere in my body, and to make sure no other tumors form in the future.

Please keep me in your thoughts during this next phase of my healing. I'm nervous, but I'm also anxious to have this large tumor gone and have a bit of peace of mind."

BRINGING MODALITIES HOME

*"My mission in life is not merely to survive, but to
thrive; and to do so with some passion, some
compassion, some humor, and some style."*
~ Maya Angelou

I returned from Germany on the evening of December 7, 2018.
I was excited to be home and to jump into all of the holiday
activities with my family!

The morning after I got home, we piled the kids into the car
and headed off to Spring Grove to chop down our Christmas
tree. This was a memory I didn't want to miss. Every year, we
take a family photo in front of the tree that we select, just before
we cut it down and haul it back to Elmhurst.

I didn't know what my future would look like – just keepin'
it real here – and although West offered to get the tree while I
was away, I knew that I *needed* to be a part of this experience.
The kids had already experienced so much change in their lives

because of this darn disease. I needed to find the energy to do this – for them, and for me.

There was also a surprise waiting for me when I returned...

"Christmas came early! I so appreciate West giving me my present, so I can continue my healing now that I've returned from Germany.

The Bemer BioMat! The same one used at Marinus.

This is one of the holistic treatments that we get daily at the Klinik. We have successfully recreated almost all of the treatments, so I can do them at home!

I am also so grateful that he manages the finances and doesn't make me stress about it. I know how incredibly expensive all of these alternative therapies are, and he's been nothing but supportive on this journey. I know he's had to get creative to cover all of these costs and make sure we still have food on the table and a roof over our heads, and that's not easy.

To learn more about the benefits of the Bemer BioMat: *www.integrativemedicine.co.za/b-e-m-e-r-therapy*"

HEADING IN THE RIGHT DIRECTION

DECEMBER 12, 2108

"Forgive yourself for not knowing what you didn't know until you lived through it.
*Honor your path. Trust your journey. Learn, grow, evolve, become." ~ **Creig Crippen***

"I had my follow up ultrasound today at Amita Cancer Center... tumor is a wee bit smaller!

Last week in Germany, the largest measurement was 4.1 cm - today the largest was 3.7 cm. It may just be margin of error, but I'm so thrilled that it seems to be heading in the right direction again. It's not growing!! Yippee! They also took blood, so I'll find out what my cancer markers are at my appointment next week."

I then had my follow up appointment with my oncologist a few days later. I was delighted to learn that the CA-15-3 cancer markers had fallen and were now back in normal range!! Maybe the treatments in Germany DID have an impact after all. Or perhaps the diet change to Keto had reversed things. Either way, I was so very grateful. I was incredibly scared for a while, but hope had now been restored.

I was gearing up for the surgery on a positive and strong note.

TOUGH CONSIDERATIONS

DECEMBER 13, 2108

"The truth is... Sometimes you have to do what's best for you and your life, not what's best for everyone else." ~ **Author Unknown**

I had my pre-op check up with my primary physician who happens to be an Integrative Medicine doctor - yes, that's the reason I chose her. It can be challenging to find medical doctors who believe in the power of FOOD. She also studied with Dr. Weil – bonus!

They swabbed my nose to check for Staph and MRSA – I've never had this done before a surgery. Glad to see they are stepping things up to avoid possible post-op infections. Thankfully everything came back clear.

She's happy about the switch to a healthy Keto approach to food, and thinks it was a good move for me at this point in the journey. My weight is stable, and my energy has increased.

She is confident that the pain and discomfort in my chest

and arm will be gone once I heal from the lumpectomy, which gives me great relief.

We discussed the possibility of having the sentinel lymph nodes removed during the surgery. It seems that the Western Medicine Doctors I speak to all follow the "standard of care," and believe that it must be done to make sure there is no spread, but I've been reading about the risks involved, and I'm not convinced that it's a necessary step for me... I must do more research, and perhaps discuss it with my surgeon to fully understand the risks and benefits.

What would I do if there are "suspicious cells" found that can't be confirmed as cancerous? This happened to a good friend of mine, and she was launched into months of chemotherapy. Would I change my treatment approach if something was found?? That was the big question...

I'm anxious to start the new year on a positive note and with more vitality!

I hope this addition to my protocol (having the tumor removed) will allow me to add a few things back into my life - like going out with friends, volunteering for the seniors, organizing events at the school (watch for a Bernie's Book Bank Book Drive coming to Emerson in the Spring), and fun adventures with my family.

MAKING TIME FOR FRIENDSHIP

"Enjoyable social interaction, community and laughter has a healing effect on the mind and body." ~ **Bryant McGill**

The value of friendship and community can't be overstated, especially during times of uncertainty. It is essential that we find a way to stay connected with those we care about, even when our worlds are turning upside down.

"A large study adds more evidence to support the power of social networks. Women diagnosed with breast cancer who had the most social ties, such as spouses, community relationships, friendships, and family members, were less likely to have the breast cancer come back (recur), and less likely to die from breast cancer than women who were socially isolated."

www.breastcancer.org/research-news/social-connections-linked-to-better-survival

My sweet friend, Sarah, organized an outing with a group of Elmhurst friends at Pinot's Palette on December 20. It was a painting party, and I even had a half glass of wine. It felt so good to get out with friends and be "normal" for a few hours!

My post to the Facebook group:

"What a fun night out with the ladies! I haven't felt very social since the diagnosis, but it truly felt great to get out with my friends for a fun evening! I needed this. Thanks for your friendship, ladies! And a special shout out to Sarah for planning such a fun night!"

TO NODE OR NOT TO NODE?

"You have the power to heal yourself, and you need to know that. We think so often that we are helpless, but we're not. We always have the power of our minds. Claim and consciously use your power."
~ Louise Hay

I had been doing a lot of research on the possible risks of having sentinel lymph nodes removed. Do I really need to do it? Is it worth the potential risks?

"Besides swelling, lymphedema also can cause arm weakness and numbness, as well as shoulder pain. Finally, the more surgery a woman has in the breast/armpit area, the more potential there is for numbness, heightened sensitivity, and discomfort."

www.breastcancer.org/treatment/surgery/lymph_node_removal/sentinel_dissection/benefits

The nurse called to schedule the lymph node procedure. I was confused... I thought the sentinel nodes were taken while the surgeon was removing the tumor, but I learned that it's actually a separate procedure, and would require a second incision.

I also learned that I needed to coordinate with the nuclear medicine department because they would be injecting a radioactive tracer to guide the surgeon to the nodes. This needed to be done prior to the scheduled surgery so it could travel to the sentinel nodes and be viewable by scan during the procedure, but doing it too early meant it might leave the body before the scan.

Ugh... I was feeling the stress build in my gut... it didn't help that, because of the timing of the tracer, I would likely need to get myself to Glenview on Christmas Eve to have it injected, since my surgery was scheduled for December 26. More time away from the family during the holidays...

So many things about this didn't feel right.

Even though they insisted that the radioactive element wasn't harmful, I was having an uncomfortable feeling about potential risks. I had been trying so hard to avoid anything that would add radiation to my body and make healing more difficult.

The nurse called me back and said that Dr. Winchester wanted to see me in person. It was amazing and impressive how much one-on-one time this busy and experienced surgeon gave me in the months prior to the surgery to make sure that my questions were answered, and I was comfortable with how we were proceeding. I still can't say enough good things about him.

AGONIZING OVER DECISIONS

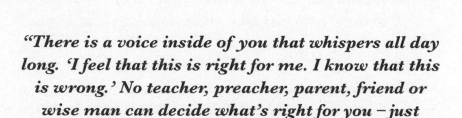

"There is a voice inside of you that whispers all day long. 'I feel that this is right for me. I know that this is wrong.' No teacher, preacher, parent, friend or wise man can decide what's right for you — just listen to the voice that speaks inside."
~ Shel Silverstein

Dr. Winchester's nurse made an appointment for December 21 so I could sit down with him and discuss removing the sentinel lymph nodes. It turned out to be a very emotional discussion, much to my surprise. I was typically very strong in my conviction, but every so often the fear got the better of me.

Dr. Winchester entered the exam room, and his calm demeanor filled the air. He had a wonderful way of supporting my wishes, yet expressing his opinion. He was always confident, but open-minded, the perfect combination for a doctor.

I turned to my list of questions:

I had read that the blue dye used for sentinel node dissection most likely will turn your skin blue, and it can last for months. This was troublesome to me – that meant something about it was remaining in my cells for quite a long time.

He said the blue dye wasn't a good option – the radioactive tracer would give us a clearer picture. I didn't like the sound of "radioactive" any more than I liked being blue. But he felt that the risks of radiation exposure were minimal, and it was necessary to use for this procedure.

"Is it possible to do the sentinel node dissection without any dye or radioactive tracer?" **no**

"What are the risks involved in having nodes removed, even just a few?" ***small chance of infection and lymphedema, as well as additional recovery time***

"If abnormal cells are found, what is the course of action?" ***Chemo***

I told him that I wasn't interested in doing Chemotherapy – if I didn't do it for a large and aggressive tumor, it wouldn't make sense to put my body through it for a suspicious node. If the testing of the node came back abnormal, I would still follow the same path of healing – the holistic approach.

He said, in so many words, that if you're not going to consider chemo, then I don't suggest you have the additional node procedure at this time. It's adding potential risks to the situation, and your recovery time will be greater. I've done a physical exam and there is no evidence of a problem with your lymph nodes, and nothing has appeared on the ultrasounds. There are no guarantees, of course, but from what we can see, there isn't a reason to worry.

I asked if this procedure could be done in the future if I suddenly began having symptoms, and he said it absolutely could. If a node becomes swollen, we could remove it at that point, and have it tested. I had elected not to have the radiation therapy after the lumpectomy, so no options would be off limits should a future problem arise (radiation may cause permanent issues with my skin, which could prevent me from having further surgeries in the future).

It felt like the right decision to avoid an additional procedure that wouldn't change my approach. Yes, the test could potentially tell me if the cancer was "on the move", but there were no signs – in my blood work, on the ultrasounds, in how I felt – that gave any indication of a problem beyond my breast. Finding a suspicious node would only create worry and stress regarding something I can't control.

He then asked if I had considered having a mastectomy – with a tumor this large, a lumpectomy would leave me deformed. I asked for more details, and he responded that he would probably be taking two thirds of my breast, but he'd do everything he could to save my nipple. He felt the tumor, and used his hands to show me a moon shape around my breast that would likely need to be removed...

Imagining what my body might look like was terrifying, and I could feel the fear bounding through my body as we spoke. I was feeling incredibly vulnerable, sitting there in a paper gown discussing my choices. Inevitably, the tears welled up in my eyes, and I began sobbing right there in front of my surgeon.

Yes, I was scared, but I knew I needed to stay true to myself and not let the fear lead me to do more than I needed. I wasn't sure how I would feel when I saw my breast after the surgery, but I felt strongly that I didn't want to jump to extreme measures like a full mastectomy if there were other reasonable options available to me.

He had been very clear that the survival rates were exactly the same for lumpectomy compared to mastectomy – it was strictly a matter of comfort level. I told him that I was certain I wanted to do the lumpectomy.

He then asked if I wanted to have reconstruction. Again, I didn't want to add any burden to my body by adding something foreign, so I declined. He assured me that we could always do reconstruction at a later date if I found it too difficult to adjust to the change of my body. It was reassuring to hear that these tough decisions weren't absolute.

And that was that. In 4 short days, I would move forward with the lumpectomy - no reconstruction, and no nodes removed.

He stood to leave, and then asked if I wanted a hug. He was kind-hearted, and could see that this was all overwhelming for me. I hugged him, thanking him for his kindness and said, "I'm sorry I make this so complicated. I must be the most difficult patient you have!"

He laughed, and said, "Not even close. We may not always agree on things, but this is your journey. We come at it from different viewpoints, but we both want what's best for you."

I feel very fortunate to have this man on my team.

"You must choose to be happy, grateful, and fulfilled. If you make that choice every single day, regardless of where you are or what's happening, you will be happy." ~ Rachel Hollis

My post to the private group:

"I got the call from the hospital today - they need me to arrive at 6 am for an 8:30 am lumpectomy at Glenbrook Hospital in Glenview.

Thankfully, my mom is an angel, and has agreed to stay overnight on Christmas and watch the kids while we're gone the following day.

If all goes well, I should be recovering for a week to 10 days. With the kids being on break from school, they would love to have play dates if anyone is in town!

Thanks, as always, for the love and support. I'm anxious and nervous about the surgery, but am so grateful to know I've got an amazing group of people sending positive healing thoughts!"

DAY OF LUMPECTOMY

DECEMBER 26, 2018

"*Once you choose hope, anything is possible.*"
~ Christopher Reeve

West's posts to the private group:

"They have declared that she is ready for surgery......now we just have to wait.....and wait......and wait......and you guessed it, wait. Procedure is at 8:30 am, assuming the surgeon gets here on time (nurse says that is pretty hit or miss). The good news is that it sounds like Leslie is first in line."

"The surgeon just came out and spoke to me. Everything went well and she will be back in her room in 5-10 minutes. He won't know if he got it all until he gets the pathology reports back. He said it would probably not be until next Wednesday due to the holidays."

"I am sitting with our patient. She is in good spirits, and believes she had a conversation with the surgeon about her Spider-Man underwear. Yes, Spider-Man.

She is very happy to have the IV out of her arm, and we

think we will be headed home shortly, assuming her blood pressure and all vitals are good.

Thanks for all of the kind words and support today! She really appreciates them."

"We have made it home! She is settled downstairs and relaxing, enjoying a cherry smoothie for a little sustenance. She is happy to see her kids and mom as they arrived home from lunch shortly after we did!"

RECOVERY

**"Your CHOICES. Your DECISIONS. Your LIFE. Live
it your way with no regrets."
~ Author Unknown**

The lumpectomy went smoothly, and I felt confident in my
decision to have the tumor removed. No regrets. The entire
experience took approximately 40 minutes from the moment I
was wheeled out of the prep room until I was back in the same
room for recovery.

They sent me home with a relatively small piece of Steri-
Strip over the incision, and internal sutures that would dissolve
on their own.

I was relieved to see that my breast didn't look much different, though that was mostly due to the swelling. In fact, there
was hardly any bruising, which was amazing after my experience with the biopsy in June that left me black and blue down
my entire right side. Clearly, this surgeon knew what he was
doing.

I could see the ink dots that formed a large circle-like figure around what used to be the tumor. I asked the surgeon about it, and he said they used ultrasound to determine how much tissue to take. It was much smaller than the area he had shown me in his office a few days prior.

My post to the private Facebook group on Thursday, December 27:

"You all are so fantastic! Keep the love coming!

I'm feeling ok so far - a pretty constant dull ache when I'm not moving, similar to the pain I had from the tumor. Of course, there's some intense pain whenever I use my right arm, which I'm trying hard not to do! Obviously, it's very sore around the incision, but it's also incredibly sore in my armpit and down my arm. Ice is my friend right now.

Finding a comfortable position for sleeping was tricky... but I'm sure it will get easier each night.

We'll get the pathology report by next Wednesday - keep the prayers coming that they got clear margins!

I'm so touched by the thoughtfulness and generosity from so many... I'm so grateful that I don't have to go through this alone. FEELING BLESSED!"

GOOD NEWS

DECEMBER 28, 2018

"Now, every time I witness a strong person, I want
to know:
What darkness did you conquer in your story?
Mountains do not rise without earthquakes."
~ Katherine MacKenett

My post to the private group:

"My phone rang this morning, and I was surprised to hear my surgeon on the other end of the line. He was calling with terrific news!

The pathology report was back and the tumor margins were CLEAR!!! Hallelujah! In conventional speak, that means "they got it all"!

I know from the tests I've had over the past several months that there are cancer cells floating in my blood and circulating in my body, so I'll need to remain focused on a healthy lifestyle so they are never given the chance to form another tumor anywhere in my body - but for now, I am OVERJOYED!! What a wonderful way to start a new year!"

I am so impressed with this amazing person, my surgeon. Of course, I expected him to do a brilliant job because of his experience and skill, but I was deeply touched that this busy man took the time to pick up the phone and call me HIMSELF to deliver the results. Of course I cried when he gave me the news... does that really surprise you?! ;)

Below are just some of the comments posted by my amazing friends and family upon hearing the news – they continue to bring tears of joy to this day. There is absolutely no question in my mind that having this incredible support system surrounding me with love has been essential to my healing.

"AMAZING news!!! SO happy to hear this!!! Happy New Year! ❤"

"Happy New Year! Happy New Year Indeed!!! Ya might just have the best night's sleep tonight than you've had in a long while :) Much love and then some to you my friend!!! Thank you for sharing this journey and this great news!! Big hugs to you and your family!"

"BEST CHRISTMAS GIFT EVER!!! So happy to hear this news!!"

"So, so thrilled to read this, Leslie!!! **XOXOXO**!!!"

. . .

"Amazing news!!! Stay the course!"

"Absolutely fantastic, Leslie!! Wishing a fast and complete recovery and return to the activities you love! Happy new year!!"

"BEST. CHRISTMAS. GIFT."

"YESSSSSS!!! Thank you for sharing this wonderful, fantastic, amazing news!"

"Great news Leslie!! And as a side note, everyone has cancer cells floating around their blood stream...it's always best to live and eat a cancer free lifestyle. Xo"

"SO THRILLED TO READ THIS NEWS!!!!!"

"Amen! Such amazing news! Enjoy every moment of the gratitude and relief you must be feeling ❤"

"Excellent news!! SO incredibly happy that you can breathe in a sigh of relief to end this year. Happy New Year!!!"

"OMG THIS IS SUCH GREAT NEWS!!!"

. . .

"Now THAT is a happy new year!"

"Wonderful news to end the year on a happy note!!"

"That makes me so happy, Lester. You are loved!!"

"Prayers answered!! Hallelujah!!! Looking forward to 2019 full of music, healthy meals, yoga and laughter with you my friend."

"Aaahhhh this is sooo incredible!!! Feeling so much gratitude for your beautiful life and your healing journey!!! Celebrating over here for you!! ❤❤❤"

THE HEALING CONTINUES

"Health does not always come from medicine. Most of the time it comes from peace of mind, peace in heart, peace in the soul. It comes from laughter and love." ~ **Author Unknown**

My post to the private group on January 5, 2019:

"I'm healing well and excited to get back to normal life! If I get the thumbs up at my post-op appointment on Wednesday, I'm planning to get my tired body to a restorative yoga class on Thursday! I can't wait to start taking care of myself again...

Thanks again to Vanessa for setting up the Meal Train for our family. The final meal was delivered last night! We all felt so loved by the nutritious food that was lovingly prepared for us and brought to our door.

A special thank you to Christy for our pot roast dinner with roasted brussels sprouts on Thursday night! The truly amazing thing is - I don't even know Christy. I haven't met her or her son, but she's a fellow mom at our school who saw Vanessa's post and wanted to help out. My heart is so touched and filled with gratitude for this stranger's kindness.

It's been a crazy roller coaster of a journey... Please know that not a single moment of kindness has slipped past me - it has all touched my heart. I've been more aware of simple kindness and love over the last half year than ever before, and I wish I could express what it has meant to me.

I couldn't have done this alone... I'm so very glad I didn't have to.

Hugs and kisses to all of you and sincere thanks for so much love and support in many forms. It is this team of amazing people that has helped me get through the last 6 months and come out stronger on the other side. So incredibly grateful for all of you!!"

POST-OP

*"The secret of health for both mind and body is not to mourn for the past, nor to worry about the future, but to live the present moment wisely and earnestly." ~ **Budha***

My post to the private Facebook group:

"I had my surgical post-op appointment today and got the all clear! The doc said I'm healing perfectly, and I can now return to my regular activities. Yoga, anyone? ☺

I'll be getting physical exams and blood tests every 3 months to make sure nothing is growing back, and to check that my nodes are still not involved. I'll also be seeing my oncologist on Jan 29 who will be a part of this monitoring process. She'll keep an eye on my liver enzymes and watch for other signs of trouble.

Hopefully I won't have anything else to report on this page! So I'll sign off for now with a HUGE amount of gratitude for the amazing support from this lovely group of people that I'm proud to call my friends.

I know in my heart that I wouldn't have gotten to this side of the journey without so many of you!! It's been a scary roller coaster of a ride for the past 6+ months, and I'm so very grateful I didn't have to ride alone. So much love to you all!!!"

MY NEW NORMAL

MARCH 23, 2019

"Joy does not simply happen to us. We have to
choose joy and keep choosing it every day."
~ Henri J.M. Nouwen

My post to the private Facebook group:

"It's been a while since my last post to this private group, so I thought I'd check in.

I have healed well from the surgery, though I've had shoulder problems ever since. I'm in PT hoping it will improve, but it's taking its sweet time. Slowly increasing range of motion and experiencing less pain.

I had a follow up with my Integrative Oncologist at the end of January. She did a physical exam and said everything looks good - scar is healing well, and the nodes feel normal as far as she can tell. They drew blood, and the results came back all in good ranges! Cancer markers are even lower than December levels.

I have been having some challenges keeping my mind from

going to dark places on occasion, especially during the quiet dark hours of the early morning - wondering if the pain in my shoulder could possibly be a sign that the cancer has spread to the bones, or if the pains around my breast could be a new tumor growing, or if my headaches are an indication that it's traveled to my brain.

I've heard these concerns are very common once you've been faced with a cancer diagnosis. I've been told it gets a bit better, but the fear never goes away completely.

I've got to find a way to recognize this fear and then let it go. If there's a reason to worry, then I will absolutely check it out and take action, but until then, I'm just worrying needlessly.

To help put my mind at ease, I requested a monitoring ultrasound of both breasts (I did have that suspicious shadow on the left), and both axilla (to check for lymph node involvement). It was once again a struggle to get it done without a mammogram, but I stood firm and they acquiesced.

We won't have official results for several weeks, but West was kind enough to accompany me, and he watched the images like a hawk! He's nearly a pro at reading sonograms by this point!

They did see what appears to be a cyst under my scar, but they weren't concerned about it.

And we were happy to see that the only suspicious shadow they could find on the left side was a mere .2 cm, so if it's the same shadow, it is now smaller! (It measured .9 cm last July, then .5 cm last September) If it is indeed cancer - well, my body is doing its job and clearing it out!

And all of my lymph nodes on both sides looked clear and healthy - a huge relief, since I opted not to have any nodes removed during my lumpectomy.

So... at this point I'm in that transition period between:

"Crap! I've got cancer... how do I make sure I don't die?!", and: "Life is rosy and everything's great!" Which looks a bit like: "Ok, so we think the cancer is gone, but you never know, and I'm not willing to do the multitude of harmful and stressful tests to search for problems, so there's no telling what's lurking"; and hopefully getting to: "I've done everything I can do to be the healthiest version of myself, and I will continue to do so in an effort to stay healthy and strong, so I need to trust in that and try to enjoy each day that I'm given."

It's a tough balancing act, but I know there are many who would be happy to be in this transition, so I'm not complaining - just trying to find my way through.

I'm slowly finding my new normal and easing back into the joy of the everyday. It's a process and I'm taking it one step at a time.

Love to you all!! XOXO"

BE THE CAPTAIN OF YOUR SHIP

"Know this one great truth: you are in control of your own life. You get one and only one chance to live." ~ **Rachel Hollis**

Something important that I learned on this journey is that, within reason, the patient should be in charge of directing their care.

They should build a team of doctors and healers who can support their chosen path, and while guidance is often necessary, the ultimate final decision-maker should always be the *patient.* It is my body and my future that we are dealing with, so I have the right to say what I'm willing to do to it.

Yes, the doctors have the medical knowledge, but they are still human, and even cancer researchers admit there is so much we don't know about cancer... so to blindly follow one person's advice without doing some reading on your own and truly understanding what is best for your individual situation just didn't feel right to me.

It may feel uncomfortable at first to question a doctor's advice, but it can also be empowering. So often, we are taught to do whatever the "man in the white coat" says we should do. I, too, had this ingrained in me, and I had to fight hard against that feeling, so I could stand in my truth.

We absolutely have the right – no, the *responsibility* – to speak up, ask questions and make final decisions that are in line with our beliefs about our own care.

I also strongly believe in getting second and third opinions, especially when it comes to big issues like a life-threatening diagnosis or potentially harmful treatments or surgery. Gathering different perspectives as well as expert advice will strengthen your knowledge base, and allow you to make the decision that is best for you.

In the end, we simply must be advocates for ourselves.

And it should be said that there is much to be learned from first-hand accounts of healing. I've learned so much from my fellow Cancer Thrivers who followed an alternative path. I am so very grateful to have the resources to connect with others around the world.

It was eye-opening to learn that there were other options out there that the surgeons and oncologists I met didn't support or perhaps even know much about. Not every therapy or approach felt right to me, but I'm glad I was able to consider each one and make the decision for myself.

Time and time again, I have found myself choosing quality over quantity. I want more life in my years - not just more years in my life.

FINAL THOUGHTS

"Be grateful for what comes next on your journey.
Be grateful for the experience. Be grateful that you
are equipped to handle it. Be grateful for what life
reveals to you. Be grateful that you are becoming
who you are meant to be. Be grateful for your
strength, your perseverance, and your courage. Be
grateful for the guiding touch from the love within."
~ Creig Crippen

I am proud of the journey I have traveled. It certainly wasn't easy, and I felt tremendous fear along the way. But as I look back over my decisions at each step, I am comforted knowing that I considered all viewpoints, did my research, talked to those who have walked before me, and made the choices that were absolutely right for ME.

I am grateful for finding Marinus, and grateful for those who led me to it. Dr. Weber is tremendous at working with you as an individual - he will offer suggestions, but he allows you to be the guide, as he strongly believes that the patient's thoughts about a treatment will affect how well the treatment works.

The mind is a very powerful tool. If you believe in what you are doing with conviction, then it is more likely to be successful. If you have doubts, then you are creating an obstacle to that success.

We've all heard of the Placebo Effect – when a patient is given a placebo (like a sugar pill or saline solution) but believes they are getting the actual treatment, and their condition improves simply because the patient had the expectation that it would help. That is the mind in action. Our thoughts create our reality.

I've met friends in Germany who did indeed do conventional treatments prior to going to Marinus, and some who had Dr. W. do their surgery onsite. I've also met a few friends who did more aggressive types of treatments there, such as low-dose chemotherapy. Dr. W. is quite open-minded, which I really appreciate. He's also open to considering new research or studies and integrating it when appropriate.

I wanted to approach my healing with baby steps - not jumping to anything harmful before fully understanding what I was doing. I wanted to see if I could heal holistically. If I had done surgery before heading to the clinic, I wouldn't have had the opportunity to measure the tumor and see firsthand what was having an effect. I was my very own science experiment.

It was terrifying, but I do believe that everything I did for 6 months leading up to the lumpectomy allowed my surgeon to get clean margins - the aggressive tumor was encapsulated and the blood vessels were limited. Hallelujah!

I strongly believe that my life would look very different right now if I had followed the conventional medicine path, and had done the triple cocktail of chemo, immediate surgery and radiation. I don't think I would feel healthy and vibrant a year after diagnosis, and I believe that I'd be struggling with long-term challenges for the rest of my life.

I've said it before, and I'll continue saying it... I AM SO GRATEFUL

AN IMPORTANT SIDE NOTE

"I am thankful for my struggle, because without it I wouldn't have stumbled across my strength."
~ Alex Elle

People often ask me if breast cancer is in my family history, and the answer is no. I do, however, have many family members on both sides who have been diagnosed with a range of different cancers (lung, thyroid, skin, kidney, prostate), as well as autoimmune diseases such as Lupus and Rheumatoid Arthritis, and serious cases of heart disease and heart attacks.

All of these are considered "lifestyle diseases", meaning diet, exercise and how we live our lives in general can have a large impact on managing these diseases.

Many doctors now believe that cancer is a chronic metabolic disease that can be managed over a lifetime. This is how I'm approaching my diagnosis going forward. The choices I make on a daily basis do indeed make a difference.

Because I understand how important it is to keep my

immune system strong in order to avoid a recurrence in the future, I've decided to head back to Marinus for maintenance treatments – I'll be leaving for Germany on July 20, 2019. I'm looking forward to boosting my health with these amazing holistic treatments to make sure any cancer cells still floating around won't ever have a chance to take hold...

I will continue visiting this healing place for maintenance once a year, and continue living the healthiest life possible as long as I am able.

Wishing you all peace, good health and lots of love.

ABOUT THE AUTHOR

Leslie Gray Robbins is a mom of two, certified health coach, motivational speaker, voiceover actor, published author, and a *Cancer Thriver*. She is hopeful that her story can help inspire others on the cancer journey to consider all options and stand in their truth.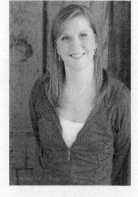

She penned her first book with her daughter Addison Baily Robbins, then 8 years old. ***What Makes A Family?*** focuses on the many ways that families are created, and can be found at Barnes & Noble and on Amazon.

Are you living your healthiest and happiest life? **Leslie** can guide you in making subtle changes in your everyday life, helping you reach your personal goals and be your BEST self.

To learn more about this side of Leslie, please visit **www.balancedlifehealthyyou.com**

In addition to being a health coach and helping people

improve their lives, **Leslie** is also a professional voiceover artist. She has had the pleasure of working with esteemed clients such as Sargento, Ghirardelli Chocolates, Capri Sun, Travelocity, Enbrel, Hampton Inn, and Blue Cross Blue Shield, among others – view her acting website at:

www.LeslieGrayRobbins.com

Leslie continues to sing whenever she gets the chance and is very grateful for her partner in crime, Carrie Marcotte, who helped created the group TAKE TWO Singers.

www.TakeTwoSingers.com

Leslie also created the a cappella group, Route 66 in 1994, and continues to make music with these amazing ladies whenever possible! Check out the tight harmonies here: **www.facebook.com/route66sings**

Made in the USA
Monee, IL
27 June 2020